**HEART&™
STROKE
FOUNDATION
OF CANADA**

Advanced Cardiovascular Life Support

P R O V I D E R   M A N U A L

Editors
Elizabeth Sinz, MD, *Associate Science Editor*
Kenneth Navarro, *Content Consultant*

Senior Managing Editor
Erik S. Soderberg, MS

Special Contributors
Clifton W. Callaway, MD, PhD
Diana M. Cave, RN, MSN
Heba Costandy, MD, MS
Mary Fran Hazinski, RN, MSN
Theresa Hoadley, RN, PhD, TNS
Robert W. Neumar, MD, PhD
Peter D. Panagos, MD
Sallie Young, PharmD, BCPS

ACLS Subcommittee 2010-2011
Clifton W. Callaway, MD, PhD, *Chair*
Robert W. Neumar, MD, PhD, *Immediate Past Chair, 2008-2010*
Steven Brooks, MD
Daniel P. Davis, MD
Michael Donnino, MD
Andrea Gabrielli, MD
Romergryko Geocadin, MD
Erik Hess, MD, MSc
Mark S. Link, MD
Bryan McNally, MD, MPH
Venu Menon, MD
Graham Nichol, MD, MPH
Brian O'Neil, MD
Joseph P. Ornato, MD
Charles W. Otto, MD
Michael Shuster, MD
Scott M. Silvers, MD
Mintu Turakhia, MD, MS
Terry L. Vanden Hoek, MD
Janice L. Zimmerman, MD

© 2011 American Heart Association
ISBN 978-1-926969-16-9
Printed in Canada
First Heart and Stroke Foundation of Canada Printing October 2011
10 9 8 7 6 5 4 3 2

ACLS Subcommittee 2009-2010

Robert W. Neumar, MD, PhD, *Chair*

Laurie J. Morrison, MD, MSc, *Immediate Past Chair, 2006-2008*

Steven Brooks, MD

Clifton W. Callaway, MD, PhD

Daniel P. Davis, MD

Andrea Gabrielli, MD

Romergryko Geocadin, MD

Richard Kerber, MD

Mark S. Link, MD

Bryan McNally, MD, MPH

Graham Nichol, MD, MPH

Brian O'Neil, MD

Joseph P. Ornato, MD

Charles Otto, MD, PhD

Michael Shuster, MD

Scott M. Silvers, MD

Terry L. Vanden Hoek, MD

Acknowledgments

Peter Oluf Anderson, MD

Ulrik Christensen, MD

Contents

Part 3
Effective Resuscitation Team Dynamics 17

Part 4
Systems of Care 25

Part 5
The ACLS Cases

33

Contents

Note on Medication Doses

Emergency cardiovascular care is a dynamic science. Advances in treatment and drug therapies occur rapidly. Readers should use the 2010 ECC Handbook to check for changes in recommended doses, indications, and contraindications.

Contents

Part 1

Course Overview

Course Description and Goal

The Advanced Cardiovascular Life Support (ACLS) Provider Course is designed for healthcare providers who either direct or participate in the management of cardiopulmonary arrest or other cardiovascular emergencies. Through didactic instruction and active participation in simulated cases, students will enhance their skills in the diagnosis and treatment of cardiopulmonary arrest, acute arrhythmia, stroke, and acute coronary syndromes (ACS).

After successful completion of this course, students will be able to apply important concepts, including:

- The Basic Life Support (BLS) Survey
- High-quality cardiopulmonary resuscitation (CPR)
- The ACLS Survey
- The ACLS algorithms
- Effective resuscitation team dynamics
- Immediate post–cardiac arrest care

The goal of the ACLS Provider Course is to improve outcomes for adult patients with cardiac arrest or other cardiopulmonary emergencies through provider training.

Course Objectives

Upon successful completion of this course students should be able to:

- Recognize and initiate early management of periarrest conditions that may result in cardiac arrest or complicate resuscitation outcome
- Demonstrate proficiency in providing BLS care, including prioritizing chest compressions and integrating automated external defibrillator (AED) use
- Recognize and manage respiratory arrest
- Recognize and manage cardiac arrest until termination of resuscitation or transfer of care, including immediate post–cardiac arrest care
- Recognize and initiate early management of ACS, including appropriate disposition
- Recognize and initiate early management of stroke, including appropriate disposition
- Demonstrate effective communication as a member or leader of a resuscitation team and recognize the impact of team dynamics on overall team performance

Course Design

To help you achieve these objectives, the ACLS Provider Course includes practice learning stations and a Megacode evaluation station.

The *practice learning stations* give you an opportunity to actively participate in a variety of learning activities, including:

- Simulated clinical scenarios
- Demonstrations by instructors or video
- Discussion and role playing
- Practice in effective resuscitation team behaviors

In these learning stations you will practice essential skills both individually and as part of a team. This course emphasizes effective team skills as a vital part of the resuscitative effort. You will have the opportunity to practice as a team member and a team leader.

At the end of the course, you will participate in a *Megacode evaluation station* to validate your achievement of the course objectives. A simulated cardiac arrest scenario will evaluate the following:

- Knowledge of core case material and skills
- Knowledge of algorithms
- Understanding of arrhythmia interpretation
- Use of appropriate basic ACLS drug therapy
- Performance as an effective team leader

Course Prerequisites and Preparation

The Heart and Stroke Foundation of Canada (HSFC) limits enrollment in the ACLS Provider Course to healthcare providers who are required to perform ACLS skills as part of their scope of practice. Participants who enter the course must have the basic knowledge and skills to participate actively with the instructor and other students.

Before the course, please read the *ACLS Provider Manual,* identify any gaps in your knowledge, and remediate those gaps by studying the applicable content in the *ACLS Provider Manual* or other supplementary resources.

The following knowledge and skills are required for successful course completion:

- BLS skills
- Electrocardiogram (ECG) rhythm interpretation for core ACLS rhythms
- Knowledge of airway management and adjuncts
- Basic ACLS drug and pharmacology knowledge
- Practical application of ACLS rhythms and drugs
- Effective resuscitation team concepts

BLS Skills

The foundation of advanced life support is strong BLS skills. HSFC requires students to have a current HSFC BLS Healthcare Provider level C card as a prerequisite to the ACLS course. *Make sure that you are proficient in BLS skills before attending the course.*

Review the CPR and AED Testing Checklist located in the Appendix.

ECG Rhythm Interpretation for Core ACLS Rhythms

The basic cardiac arrest and periarrest algorithms require students to recognize these ECG rhythms:

- Sinus rhythm
- Atrial fibrillation and flutter
- Bradycardia
- Tachycardia
- Atrioventricular (AV) block
- Asystole
- Pulseless electrical activity (PEA)
- Ventricular tachycardia (VT)
- Ventricular fibrillation (VF)

During the course you must be able to identify and interpret rhythms during practice as well as during the final Megacode evaluation station.

Basic ACLS Drug and Pharmacology Knowledge

You must know the drugs and doses used in the ACLS algorithms. You will also need to know *when* to use *which* drug based on the clinical situation.

Effective Resuscitation Team Concepts

Instructors throughout the course will evaluate your effectiveness as a team leader and a team member. A clear understanding of these concepts is integral to successful performance in the learning activities and the Megacode test. Review Part 3 in the *ACLS Provider Manual* before the course. During the Megacode the instructor will evaluate your team leader skills with a major emphasis on your ability to direct the integration of BLS and ACLS activities by your team members.

Course Materials

Course materials consist of the *ACLS Provider Manual,* ACLS Written Precourse Self-Assessment exam, 2 pocket reference cards, and Precourse Preparation Checklist.

ACLS Provider Manual

The *ACLS Provider Manual* contains the basic information you need for effective participation in the course. This important material includes the systematic approach to a cardiopulmonary emergency, effective resuscitation team communication, and the ACLS cases and algorithms. *Please review this manual before attending the course. Bring it with you for use and reference during the course.*

The manual is organized into the following parts:

		Contents
Part 1	Course Overview	
Part 2	The Systematic Approach	
Part 3	Effective Resuscitation Team Dynamics	
Part 4	Systems of Care	
Part 5	The ACLS Cases	
Appendix		
• **Testing Checklists and Learning Station Checklists**		
• ***2010 Guidelines for CPR and ECC Summary Table***	Summary of the new *2010 Guidelines for CPR and ECC*	
• **ACLS Pharmacology Summary Table**	Basic ACLS drugs, doses, indications/contraindications, and side effects	
• **Glossary**	Alphabetical list of terms	
• **Foundation Index**	Pages where key subjects can be found (e.g., epinephrine, cardioversion, pacing)	
Index		

HSFC strongly recommends that students complete the Written Precourse Self-Assessment exam available from the Course Administrator and bring their scores for discussion with their ACLS Instructor.

Call-out Boxes

The *ACLS Provider Manual* contains important information presented in call-out boxes that require the reader's attention. Please pay particular attention to the call-out boxes, listed below:

- Critical Concepts
- Caution
- FYI 2010 Guidelines
- Foundational Facts

Critical Concepts **Important Information to Review and Study**	• Pay particular attention to the **Critical Concepts** boxes that appear in the *ACLS Provider Manual*. These boxes contain the most important information that you must know.

| **Caution** | • **Caution** boxes emphasize specific risks associated with interventions. |

| **FYI 2010 Guidelines** | • **FYI 2010 Guidelines** boxes contain the new *2010 Guidelines for CPR and ECC* information. |

| **Foundational Facts** | • You will see **Foundational Facts** boxes throughout the *ACLS Provider Manual*. These boxes contain basic information that will help you understand the topics covered in the course. |

Pocket Reference Cards

The Pocket Reference Cards are 2 stand-alone cards packaged with the *ACLS Provider Manual.* These cards can be carried in your pocket for quick reference on the following topics:

Topic	Reference Cards
Cardiac arrest, arrhythmias, and treatment	• Cardiac Arrest Algorithms • Gray box with drugs and dosage reminders • Immediate Post–Cardiac Arrest Care Algorithm • Bradycardia Algorithm • Tachycardia Algorithm
ACS and stroke	• ACS Algorithm • Fibrinolytic Checklist for STEMI • Fibrinolytic Contraindications for STEMI • Suspected Stroke Algorithm • Stroke Assessment–CPSS • Use of IV rtPA for Acute Ischemic Stroke • Hypertension Management in Acute Ischemic Stroke

Precourse Preparation Checklist

The Precourse Preparation Checklist is packaged with the *ACLS Provider Manual.* Please review and check the boxes after you have completed preparation for each section.

Requirements for Successful Course Completion

To successfully complete the ACLS Provider Course and obtain your course completion card, you must:

- Pass the 1-Rescuer Adult CPR and AED Test
- Pass the Bag-Mask Ventilation Test
- Demonstrate competency in learning station skills
- Pass the Megacode Test
- Pass the closed-book written exam with a minimum score of 84%

ACLS Update Course

The ACLS Update Course is for students who have a current ACLS Provider card and need to update and refresh their ACLS skills. This course is primarily focused on skills competency testing.

- Maximum renewal period: 2 years
- Update requirements: Previous ACLS course completion card (not expired)

ACLS Provider Manual Abbreviations

A	
ABCD	ACLS Survey: Airway, Breathing, Circulation, Differential Diagnosis
ACE	Angiotensin-converting enzyme
ACLS	Advanced cardiovascular life support
ACS	Acute coronary syndromes
AED	Automated external defibrillator
AHF	Acute heart failure
AIVR	Accelerated idioventricular rhythm
AMI	Acute myocardial infarction
aPTT	Activated partial thromboplastin time
B	
BLS	Basic life support: Check responsiveness, activate emergency response system, check carotid pulse, provide defibrillation
C	
CARES	Cardiac Arrest Registry to Enhance Survival
CPR	Cardiopulmonary resuscitation
CPSS	Cincinnati Prehospital Stroke Scale
CT	Computed tomography

(continued)

(continued)

D	
DNAR	Do not attempt resuscitation

E	
ECG	Electrocardiogram
ED	Emergency department
EMS	Emergency medical services
ET	Endotracheal

F	
FDA	Food and Drug Administration
FIO₂	Fraction of inspired oxygen

G	
GI	Gastrointestinal

I	
ICU	Intensive care unit
INR	International normalized ratio
IO	Intraosseous
IV	Intravenous

L	
LMWH	Low-molecular-weight heparin
LV	Left ventricle or left ventricular

M	
mA	Milliamperes
MACE	Major adverse cardiac events
MET	Medical emergency team
MI	Myocardial infarction
mm Hg	Millimeters of mercury

N	
NIH	National Institutes of Health
NIHSS	National Institutes of Health Stroke Scale
NINDS	National Institute of Neurological Disorders and Stroke
NPA	Nasopharyngeal airway
NSAIDs	Nonsteroidal anti-inflammatory drugs
NSTEMI	Non–ST-segment elevation myocardial infarction

(continued)

(continued)

O	
OPA	Oropharyngeal airway

P	
$Paco_2$	Partial pressure of carbon dioxide in arterial blood
PCI	Percutaneous coronary intervention
PE	Pulmonary embolism
PEA	Pulseless electrical activity
PT	Prothrombin time

R	
ROSC	Return of spontaneous circulation
RRT	Rapid response team
rtPA	Recombinant tissue plasminogen activator
RV	Right ventricle or right ventricular

S	
SBP	Systolic blood pressure
STEMI	ST-segment elevation myocardial infarction
SVT	Supraventricular tachycardia

T	
TCP	Transcutaneous pacing

U	
UA	Unstable angina
UFH	Unfractionated heparin

V	
VF	Ventricular fibrillation
VT	Ventricular tachycardia

Part 2

The Systematic Approach: The BLS and ACLS Surveys

Introduction

Healthcare providers use a systematic approach to assess and treat arrest and acutely ill or injured patients for optimum care. The goal of the resuscitation team's interventions for a patient in respiratory or cardiac arrest is to support and restore effective oxygenation, ventilation, and circulation with return of intact neurologic function. An intermediate goal of resuscitation is the return of spontaneous circulation (ROSC). The actions used are guided by the following systematic approaches:

- BLS Survey (steps designated by the numbers 1, 2, 3, 4)
- ACLS Survey (steps designated by the letters A, B, C, D)

Learning Objectives

By the end of this part you should be able to:

1. Describe the critical actions of the BLS Survey and ACLS Survey

2. Describe assessment and management that occur with each step of the systematic approach

3. Describe how the assessment/management approach is applicable to most cardio-pulmonary emergencies

The Systematic Approach: The BLS and ACLS Surveys

Overview of the Systematic Approach

The systematic approach first requires ACLS providers to determine the patient's level of consciousness. As you approach the patient:

- If the patient appears unconscious
  - Use the BLS Survey for the initial assessment.
  - After completing all of the appropriate steps of the BLS Survey, use the ACLS Survey for more advanced assessment and treatment.
- If the patient appears conscious
  - Use the ACLS Survey for your initial assessment.

The details of the BLS and ACLS Surveys are described below.

The BLS Survey

Overview of the BLS Survey

The BLS Survey is a systematic approach to basic life support that any trained healthcare provider can perform. This approach stresses *early CPR* and *early defibrillation*. It does not include advanced interventions, such as advanced airway techniques or drug administration. By using the BLS Survey, healthcare providers may achieve their goal of supporting or restoring effective oxygenation, ventilation, and circulation until ROSC or initiation of ACLS interventions. Performing the actions in the BLS Survey substantially improves the patient's chance of survival and a good neurologic outcome.

Before conducting the BLS or ACLS Survey, look to make sure the scene is safe.

- The BLS Survey uses a series of 4 sequential assessment steps designated by the numbers 1, 2, 3, and 4. Simultaneously with each assessment step, you should perform appropriate corrective action(s) before proceeding to the next step. Assessment is a key component in this approach (e.g., check the pulse before starting chest compressions or attaching an AED).

> **Remember: Assess...then perform appropriate action.**

FYI 2010 Guidelines

Changes in the BLS Survey

Please note the 2 key changes from the *2005 Guidelines for CPR and ECC:*

- *The 2010 Guidelines for CPR and ECC* alters the BLS sequence by eliminating "look, listen, and feel" followed by 2 rescue breaths. This change promotes earlier initiation of chest compressions in cardiac arrest patients.
- The BLS Survey is no longer represented by the letters A, B, C, D but is represented by the numbers 1, 2, 3, 4 instead.

Foundational Facts

Starting With Chest Compressions vs 2 Breaths

- Although no published human or animal evidence demonstrates that starting CPR with 30 compressions rather than 2 ventilations leads to improved outcomes, it is clear that blood flow depends on chest compressions. Therefore, providers must minimize delays in and interruptions of chest compressions throughout the entire resuscitation. Positioning the head, achieving a seal for mouth-to-mouth rescue breaths, or getting a bag-mask device for rescue breaths takes time. Beginning CPR with 30 compressions rather than 2 ventilations leads to a shorter delay to the first compression.
- Once one provider begins chest compressions, a second trained healthcare provider should deliver rescue breaths to provide oxygenation and ventilation as follows:
  - Deliver each rescue breath over 1 second
  - Give a sufficient tidal volume to produce visible chest rise

Although the BLS Survey requires no advanced equipment, healthcare providers can use any readily available universal precaution supplies or adjuncts, such as a bag-mask ventilation device. Whenever possible, place the patient on a firm surface in a supine position to maximize the effectiveness of chest compressions. Table 1 is an overview of the BLS Survey, and Figures 1 through 4 illustrate the steps needed during the BLS Survey. Before approaching the patient, ensure scene safety.

For more details, review the VF Treated With CPR and AED Case in Part 5 of this manual.

Table 1. The BLS Survey

	Assess	Assessment Technique and Action	
1	**Check responsive-ness**	• Tap and shout, ***"Are you all right?"*** • Check for absent or abnormal breathing (no breathing or only gasping) by looking at or **scanning the chest for movement** (about 5 to 10 seconds)	 **Figure 1.** Check responsiveness.
2	**Activate the emergency response system/get AED**	• Activate the emergency response system and get an AED if one is available or send someone to activate the emergency response system and get an AED or defibrillator	 **Figure 2.** Activate the emergency response system.

3	**Circulation**	• **Check the carotid pulse** for 5 to 10 seconds
		• If no pulse within 10 seconds, start CPR (30:2) beginning with chest compressions
		  – Compress the center of the chest (lower half of the sternum) hard and fast with at least 100 compressions per minute at a depth of at least 5 cm (2 inches)
		  – Allow complete chest recoil after each compression
		  – Minimize interruptions in compressions (10 seconds or less)
		  – Switch providers about every 2 minutes to avoid fatigue
		  – Avoid excessive ventilation
		• If there is a pulse, start rescue breathing at 1 breath every 5 to 6 seconds (10 to 12 breaths per minute). Check pulse about every 2 minutes
			
			Figure 3. Check the carotid pulse.

4	**Defibrillation**	• If no pulse, check for a shockable rhythm with an AED/defibrillator as soon as it arrives • Provide shocks as indicated • Follow each shock immediately with CPR, beginning with compressions	 **Figure 4.** Defibrillation.

Critical Concepts Minimizing Interruptions	**ACLS providers must make every effort to minimize any interruptions in chest compressions.** Try to limit interruptions in chest compressions (e.g., defibrillation and advanced airway) to no longer than 10 seconds, except in extreme circumstances, such as removing the patient from a dangerous environment. When you stop chest compressions, blood flow to the brain and heart stops. **Avoid:** • Prolonged rhythm analysis • Frequent or inappropriate pulse checks • Taking too long to give breaths to the patient • Unnecessarily moving the patient

Foundational Facts Lone Healthcare Provider May Tailor Response	• Lone healthcare providers may tailor the sequence of rescue actions to the most likely cause of arrest. For example, if a lone healthcare provider sees an adolescent suddenly collapse, it is reasonable to assume that the patient has suffered a sudden cardiac arrest. • The lone rescuer should call for help (activate the emergency response system), get an AED (if nearby), return to the patient to attach the AED, and then provide CPR. • On the other hand, if hypoxia is the presumed cause of the cardiac arrest (such as in a drowning patient), the healthcare provider may give about 5 cycles (approximately 2 minutes) of CPR before activating the emergency response system.

Critical Concepts High-Quality CPR	• Compress the chest hard and fast. • Allow complete chest recoil after each compression. • Minimize interruptions in compressions (10 seconds or less). • Switch providers about every 2 minutes to avoid fatigue. • Avoid excessive ventilation.

The ACLS Survey

Overview of the ACLS Survey

For unconscious patients in arrest (cardiac or respiratory):

• Healthcare providers should conduct the ACLS Survey after completing the BLS survey.

For conscious patients who may need more advanced assessment and management techniques:

• Healthcare providers should conduct the ACLS Survey first.

An important component of this survey is the differential diagnosis, where identification and treatment of the underlying causes may be critical to patient outcome.

In the ACLS Survey you continue to assess and perform an action as appropriate until transfer to the next level of care. Many times, team members perform assessments and actions in ACLS simultaneously.

Remember: Assess...then perform appropriate action.

Table 2 provides an overview of the ACLS Survey. The ACLS cases provide details on these components.

Table 2. The ACLS Survey

Assess	Action as Appropriate

Airway
 	
- *Is the airway patent?*
- *Is an advanced airway indicated?*
- *Is proper placement of airway device confirmed?*
- *Is tube secured and placement reconfirmed frequently?*
	• **Maintain airway patency in unconscious patients** by use of the head tilt–chin lift, oropharyngeal airway (OPA), or nasopharyngeal airway (NPA)
	• **Use advanced airway management if needed** (e.g.,laryngeal mask airway, laryngeal tube, esophageal-tracheal tube, endotracheal tube [ET tube])
	
	Healthcare providers must weigh the benefit of advanced airway placement against the adverse effects of interrupting chest compressions. If bag-mask ventilation is adequate, healthcare providers may defer insertion of an advanced airway until the patient fails to respond to initial CPR and defibrillation or until spontaneous circulation returns. Advanced airway devices such as a laryngeal mask airway, laryngeal tube, or esophageal-tracheal tube can be placed while chest compressions continue.
	
	If using advanced airway devices:
	
	• **Confirm proper integration of CPR and ventilation**
	• **Confirm proper placement of advanced airway devices** by
	  – Physical examination
	  – Quantitative waveform capnography
	    ▪ Class I recommendation for ET tube
	    ▪ Reasonable for supraglottic airways
	• **Secure the device to prevent dislodgment**
	• **Monitor airway placement with continuous quantitative waveform capnography**

Breathing
 	
- *Are ventilation and oxygenation adequate?*
- *Are quantitative waveform capnography and oxyhemoglobin saturation monitored?*
	• **Give supplementary oxygen when indicated**
	  – For cardiac arrest patients, administer 100% oxygen
	  – For others, titrate oxygen administration to achieve oxygen saturation values of ≥94% by pulse oximetry
	• **Monitor the adequacy of ventilation and oxygenation** by
	  – Clinical criteria (chest rise and cyanosis)
	  – Quantitative waveform capnography
	  – Oxygen saturation
	• **Avoid excessive ventilation**

(continued)

(continued)

Assess	Action as Appropriate

Circulation
 	
– *Are chest compressions effective?*
– *What is the cardiac rhythm?*
– *Is defibrillation or cardioversion indicated?*
– *Has IV/IO access been established?*
– *Is ROSC present?*
– *Is the patient with a pulse unstable?*
– *Are medications needed for rhythm or blood pressure?*
– *Does the patient need volume (fluid) for resuscitation?*
	• **Monitor CPR quality**
	  – Quantitative waveform capnography (if $P_{ET}CO_2$ is <10 mm Hg, attempt to improve CPR quality)
	  – Intra-arterial pressure (if relaxation phase [diastolic] pressure is <20 mm Hg, attempt to improve CPR quality)
	• **Attach monitor/defibrillator for arrhythmias or cardiac arrest rhythms** (e.g., VF, pulseless VT, asystole, PEA)
	• **Provide defibrillation/cardioversion**
	• **Obtain IV/IO access**
	• **Give appropriate drugs** to manage rhythm and blood pressure
	• **Give IV/IO fluids if needed**

Differential diagnosis – *Why did this patient develop symptoms or arrest?* – *Is there a reversible cause that can be treated?*	• **Search for, find, and treat reversible causes** (i.e., definitive care)

$P_{ET}CO_2$ is the partial pressure of CO_2 in exhaled air at the end of the exhalation phase.

Effective Resuscitation Team Dynamics

Introduction

Successful resuscitation attempts often require healthcare providers to simultaneously perform a variety of interventions. Although a CPR-trained bystander working alone can resuscitate a patient within the first moments after collapse, most attempts require the concerted efforts of multiple healthcare providers. Effective teamwork divides the tasks while multiplying the chances of a successful outcome.

Successful teams not only have medical expertise and mastery of resuscitation skills, but they also demonstrate effective communication and team dynamics. Part 3 of this manual discusses the importance of team roles, behaviors of effective team leaders and team members, and elements of effective resuscitation team dynamics.

During the course you will have an opportunity to practice performing different roles as a member and a leader of a simulated resuscitation team.

Learning Objectives

By the end of this part you should be able to:

1. Describe team leader's and team members' roles

2. Explain the importance of the team leader and team members understanding their specific roles

3. Describe how skills mastery combined with team dynamics may lead to increased success in resuscitation outcomes

4. Describe key elements of an effective resuscitation

5. Coordinate team functions while ensuring continuous high-quality CPR, defibrillation, and rhythm assessment

Foundational Facts
Understanding Team Roles

Whether you are a team member or team leader during a resuscitation attempt, you should **understand not only your role but also the roles of other team members.** This awareness will help you anticipate:

- What actions will be performed next
- How to communicate and work as a member or leader of the team

Roles of the Team Leader and Team Members

Role of the Team Leader

The role of the team leader is multifaceted. The team leader:

- Organizes the group
- Monitors individual performance of team members
- Backs up team members
- Models excellent team behavior
- Trains and coaches
- Facilitates understanding
- Focuses on comprehensive patient care

Every resuscitation team needs a leader to organize the efforts of the group. The team leader is responsible for making sure everything is done at the right time in the right way by monitoring and integrating individual performance of team members. The role of the team leader is similar to that of an orchestra conductor directing individual musicians. Like a conductor, the team leader does not play the instruments but instead knows how each member of the orchestra fits into the overall music.

The role of the team leader also includes modeling excellent team behavior and leadership skills for the team and other people involved or interested in the resuscitation. The team leader should serve as a teacher or guide to help train future team leaders and improve team effectiveness. After resuscitation the team leader can facilitate analysis, critique, and practice in preparation for the next resuscitation attempt.

The team leader also helps team members understand why they must perform certain tasks in a specific way. The team leader should be able to explain why it is essential to:

- Push hard and fast
- Ensure complete chest recoil
- Minimize interruptions in chest compressions
- Avoid excessive ventilations

Whereas team members should focus on their individual tasks, the team leader must focus on comprehensive patient care.

Role of the Team Member

Team members must be proficient in performing the skills authorized by their scope of practice. It is essential to the success of the resuscitation attempt that team members are:

- Clear about role assignments
- Prepared to fulfill their role responsibilities
- Well practiced in resuscitation skills
- Knowledgeable about the algorithms
- Committed to success

Elements of Effective Resuscitation Team Dynamics

Closed-Loop Communications

When communicating with resuscitation team members, the team leader should use closed-loop communication by taking these steps:

1. The team leader gives a message, order, or assignment to a team member.

2. By receiving a clear response and eye contact, the team leader confirms that the team member heard and understood the message.

3. The team leader listens for confirmation of task performance from the team member before assigning another task.

Do

Team leader	• Assign another task after receiving oral confirmation that a task has been completed, such as, "Now that the IV is in, give 1 mg of epinephrine"
Team members	• Close the loop: Inform the team leader when a task begins or ends, such as, "The IV is in"

Don't

Team leader	• Give more tasks to a team member without asking or receiving confirmation of a completed assignment
Team members	• Give drugs without verbally confirming the order with the team leader • Forget to inform the team leader after giving the drug or performing the procedure

Clear Messages

Clear messages consist of concise communication spoken with distinctive speech in a controlled tone of voice. All healthcare providers should deliver messages and orders in a calm and direct manner without yelling or shouting. Unclear communication can lead to unnecessary delays in treatment or to medication errors.

For example: "Did the patient get IV propofol so I can proceed with the cardioversion?" "No, I thought you said to give him propranolol."

Yelling or shouting can impair effective team interaction. Only one person should talk at any time.

Do

Team leader	• Encourage team members to speak clearly
Team members	• Repeat the medication order • Question an order if the slightest doubt exists

Don't

Team leader	• Mumble or speak in incomplete sentences • Give unclear messages and drug/medication orders • Yell, scream, or shout
Team members	• Feel patronized by distinct and concise messages

Clear Roles and Responsibilities

Every member of the team should know his or her role and responsibilities. Just as different shaped pieces make up a jigsaw puzzle, each team member's role is unique and critical to the effective performance of the team. Figure 5 identifies 6 team roles for resuscitation. When <6 people are present, all tasks must be assigned to the healthcare providers present.

When roles are unclear, team performance suffers. Signs of unclear roles include:

- Performing the same task more than once
- Missing essential tasks
- Freelancing of team members

To avoid inefficiencies, the team leader must clearly delegate tasks. Team members should communicate when and if they can handle additional responsibilities. The team leader should encourage team members to participate in leadership and not simply follow directions blindly.

Do

Team leader	• Clearly define all team member roles in the clinical setting
Team members	• Seek out and perform clearly defined tasks appropriate to your level of competence • Ask for a new task or role if you are unable to perform your assigned task because it is beyond your level of experience or competence

Don't

Team leader	• Neglect to assign tasks to all available team members • Assign tasks to team members who are unsure of their responsibilities • Distribute assignments unevenly, leaving some with too much to do and others with too little
Team members	• Avoid taking assignments • Take assignments beyond your level of competence or expertise

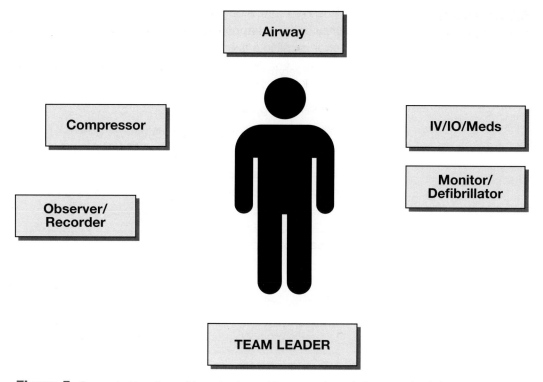

Figure 5. Suggested locations of team leader and team members during case simulations.

Knowing One's Limitations

Not only should everyone on the team know his or her own limitations and capabilities, but the team leader should also be aware of them. This allows the team leader to evaluate team resources and call for backup of team members when assistance is needed. Team members should anticipate situations in which they might require assistance and inform the team leader.

During the stress of an attempted resuscitation, do not practice or explore a new skill. If you need extra help, request it early. It is not a sign of weakness or incompetence to ask for help; it is better to have more help than needed rather than not enough help, which might negatively affect patient outcome.

Do

Team leader and team members	• Call for assistance early rather than waiting until the patient deteriorates to the point that help is critical • Seek advice from more experienced personnel when the patient's condition worsens despite primary treatment

Don't

Team leader and team members	• Reject offers from others to carry out an assigned task you are unable to complete, especially if task completion is essential to treatment
Team members	• Use or start an unfamiliar treatment or therapy without seeking advice from more experienced personnel • Take on too many assignments at a time when assistance is readily available

Knowledge Sharing

Sharing information is a critical component of effective team performance. Team leaders may become trapped in a specific treatment or diagnostic approach; this common human error is called a fixation error. Examples of 3 common types of fixation errors are:

- "Everything is okay."
- "This and only this is the correct path."
- "Anything but this."

When resuscitative efforts are ineffective, go back to the basics and talk as a team. "Well, we've gotten the following on the ACLS Survey…. Have we missed something?"

Team members should inform the team leader of any changes in the patient's condition to ensure that decisions are made with all available information.

Do

Team leader	• Encourage an environment of information sharing and ask for suggestions if uncertain of the next best interventions • Ask for good ideas for differential diagnoses • Ask if anything has been overlooked (e.g., IV access should have been obtained or drugs should have been administered)
Team members	• Share information with other team members

Don't

Team leader	• Ignore others' suggestions for treatment • Overlook or fail to examine clinical signs that are relevant to the treatment
Team members	• Ignore important information to improve your role

Constructive Intervention

During a resuscitation attempt the team leader or a team member may need to intervene if an action that is about to occur may be inappropriate at the time. Although constructive intervention is necessary, it should be tactful. Team leaders should avoid confrontation with team members. Instead, conduct a debriefing afterward if constructive criticism is needed.

Do

Team leader	• Ask that a different intervention be started if it has a higher priority
Team members	• Suggest an alternative drug or dose in a confident manner • Question a colleague who is about to make a mistake

Don't

Team leader	• Fail to reassign a team member who is trying to function beyond his or her level of skill
Team members	• Ignore a team member who is about to administer a drug incorrectly

Reevaluation and Summarizing

An essential role of the team leader is monitoring and reevaluating:

- The patient's status
- Interventions that have been performed
- Assessment findings

A good practice is for the team leader to summarize this information out loud in a periodic update to the team. Review the status of the resuscitation attempt and announce the plan for the next few steps. Remember that the patient's condition can change. Remain flexible to changing treatment plans and revisiting the initial differential diagnosis. Ask for information and summaries from the code recorder as well.

Do

Team leader	• Draw continuous attention to decisions about differential diagnoses • Review or maintain an ongoing record of drugs and treatments administered and the patient's response
Team leader and team members	• Clearly draw attention to significant changes in the patient's clinical condition • Increase monitoring (e.g., frequency of respirations and blood pressure) when the patient's condition deteriorates

Don't

Team leader	• Fail to change a treatment strategy when new information supports such a change • Fail to inform arriving personnel of the current status and plans for further action

Mutual Respect

The best teams are composed of members who share a mutual respect for each other and work together in a collegial, supportive manner. To have a high-performing team, everyone must abandon ego and respect each other during the resuscitation attempt, regardless of any additional training or experience that the team leader or specific team members may have.

Do

Team leader and team members	• Speak in a friendly, controlled tone of voice • Avoid shouting or displaying aggression if you are not understood initially
Team leader	• Acknowledge correctly completed assignments by saying, "Thanks—good job!"

Don't

Team leader and team members	• Shout or yell at team members—when one person raises his voice, others will respond similarly • Behave aggressively or confuse directive behavior with aggression • Be uninterested in others

Part 4

Systems of Care

Introduction

A system is a group of regularly interacting and interdependent components. The system provides the links for the chain and determines the strength of each link and the chain as a whole. By definition, the system determines the ultimate outcome and strength of the chain and provides collective support and organization. For patients with possible ACS, the system rapidly triages patients, determines a possible or provisional diagnosis, and initiates a strategy based on initial clinical characteristics.

Learning Objectives

By the end of this part you should be able to:

1. Describe how systems of care are coordinated on the basis of the individual's health needs

2. Define systems of care that provide early access to coronary angiography, postarrest therapeutic hypothermia, and admission to units providing specialized care

3. Describe the components of a rapid response system

4. Discuss how the use of a rapid response team (RRT) or medical emergency team (MET) may improve patient outcomes

---

Cardiopulmonary Resuscitation

Quality Improvement in Resuscitation Systems, Processes, and Outcomes

Cardiopulmonary resuscitation is a series of lifesaving actions that improve the chance of survival following cardiac arrest. Although the optimal approach to CPR may vary, depending on the rescuer, the patient, and the available resources, the fundamental challenge remains how to achieve early and effective CPR.

A Systems Approach

Successful resuscitation following cardiac arrest requires an integrated set of coordinated actions represented by the links in the adult Chain of Survival (Figure 6). The links include the following:

- Immediate recognition of cardiac arrest and activation of the emergency response system
- Early CPR with an emphasis on chest compressions
- Rapid defibrillation
- Effective advanced life support
- Integrated post–cardiac arrest care

Effective resuscitation requires an integrated response known as a system of care. Fundamental to a successful resuscitation system of care is the collective appreciation of the challenges and opportunities presented by the Chain of Survival. Thus, individuals and groups must work together, sharing ideas and information, to evaluate and improve their resuscitation system. Leadership and accountability are important components of this team approach.

To improve care, leaders must assess the performance of each system component. Only when performance is evaluated can participants in a system effectively intervene to improve care. This process of quality improvement consists of an iterative and continuous cycle of:

- Systematic evaluation of resuscitation care and outcome
- Benchmarking with stakeholder feedback
- Strategic efforts to address identified deficiencies

Figure 6. The adult Chain of Survival.

Foundational Facts

Medical Emergency Teams (METs) and Rapid Response Teams (RRTs)

- Many hospitals have implemented the use of METs or RRTs. The purpose of these teams is to improve patient outcomes by identifying and treating early clinical deterioration (Figure 7). In-hospital cardiac arrest is commonly preceded by physiologic changes. In one study nearly 80% of hospitalized patients with cardiorespiratory arrest had abnormal vital signs documented for up to 8 hours before the actual arrest. Many of these changes can be recognized by monitoring routine vital signs. Intervention before clinical deterioration or cardiac arrest may be possible.
- Consider this question: "Would you have done anything differently if you knew 15 minutes before the arrest that...?"

Figure 7. Management of life-threatening emergencies requires integration of multidisciplinary teams that can involve rapid response teams, cardiac arrest teams, and intensive care specialties to achieve survival of the patient. Team leaders have an essential role in coordination of care with team members and other specialists.

Measurement

Quality improvement relies on valid assessment of resuscitation performance and outcome.

- The Utstein Guidelines provide guidance for core performance measures, including:
  - Rate of bystander CPR
  - Time to defibrillation
  - Survival to hospital discharge
- Importance of information sharing among all links in the system of care:
  - Dispatch records
  - Emergency medical services (EMS) patient care report
  - Hospital records

Change

Simply measuring and benchmarking care can positively influence outcome. However, ongoing review and interpretation are necessary to identify areas for improvement, such as:

- Increased bystander CPR response rates
- Improved CPR performance
- Shortened time to defibrillation
- Citizen awareness
- Citizen and healthcare professional education and training

Summary

Over the past 50 years the modern-era basic life support fundamentals of early recognition and activation, early CPR, and early defibrillation have saved hundreds of thousands of lives around the world. However, we still have a long road to travel if we are to fulfill the potential offered by the Chain of Survival. Survival disparities present a generation ago appear to persist. Fortunately, we currently possess the knowledge and tools—represented by the Chain of Survival—to address many of these care gaps, and future discoveries will offer opportunities to improve rates of survival.

Post–Cardiac Arrest Care

The healthcare system should implement a comprehensive, structured, multidisciplinary system of care in a consistent manner for the treatment of post–cardiac arrest patients. Programs should address therapeutic hypothermia, hemodynamic and ventilation optimization, immediate coronary reperfusion with percutaneous coronary intervention (PCI), glycemic control, neurologic care and prognostication, and other structured interventions.

Individual hospitals with a high frequency of treating cardiac arrest patients show an increased likelihood of survival when these interventions are provided.

Therapeutic Hypothermia

The *2010 Guidelines for CPR and ECC* recommends cooling comatose (i.e., lack of meaningful response to verbal commands) adult patients with ROSC after out-of-hospital VF cardiac arrest to 32°C to 34°C (89.6°F to 93.2°F) for 12 to 24 hours. Healthcare providers should also consider induced hypothermia for comatose adult patients with ROSC after in-hospital cardiac arrest of any initial rhythm or after out-of-hospital cardiac arrest with an initial rhythm of PEA or asystole.

Hemodynamic and Ventilation Optimization

Although providers often use 100% oxygen while performing the initial resuscitation, providers should titrate inspired oxygen during the post–cardiac arrest phase to the lowest level required to achieve an arterial oxygen saturation of ≥94%. This helps to avoid any potential complications associated with oxygen toxicity.

Avoid excessive ventilation of the patient because of potential adverse hemodynamic effects when intrathoracic pressures are increased and because of potential decreases in cerebral blood flow when $PaCO_2$ decreases.

Healthcare providers may start ventilation rates at 10 to 12 breaths per minute and titrate to achieve a $PETCO_2$ of 35 to 40 mm Hg or a $PaCO_2$ of 40 to 45 mm Hg.

Healthcare providers should titrate fluid administration and vasoactive or inotropic agents as needed to optimize blood pressure, cardiac output, and systemic perfusion. The optimal post–cardiac arrest blood pressure remains unknown; however, a mean arterial pressure ≥65 mm Hg is a reasonable goal.

Immediate Coronary Reperfusion With PCI

Following ROSC, rescuers should transport the patient to a facility capable of reliably providing coronary reperfusion (e.g., PCI) and other goal-directed postarrest care therapies. The decision to perform PCI can be made irrespective of the presence of coma or the decision to induce hypothermia, because concurrent PCI and hypothermia are reported to be feasible and safe and have good outcomes.

Glycemic Control

Consider strategies to target moderate glycemic control (144 to 180 mg/dL [8 to 10 mmol/L]) in adult patients with ROSC after cardiac arrest.

Healthcare providers should not attempt to alter glucose concentration within a lower range (80 to 110 mg/dL [4.4 to 6.1 mmol/L]) due to the increased risk of hypoglycemia.

Neurologic Care and Prognostication

The goal of post–cardiac arrest management is to return patients to their prearrest functional level. Reliable early prognostication of neurologic outcome is an essential component of post–cardiac arrest care. Most importantly, when considering decisions to limit or withdraw life-sustaining care, tools used to prognosticate poor outcome must be accurate and reliable, with a false-positive rate approaching 0%.

Acute Coronary Syndromes

The primary goals of therapy for patients with ACS are to:

1. Reduce the amount of myocardial necrosis that occurs in patients with acute myocardial infarction (AMI), thus preserving left ventricular (LV) function, preventing heart failure, and limiting other cardiovascular complications

2. Prevent major adverse cardiac events (MACE): death, nonfatal MI, and the need for urgent revascularization

3. Treat acute, life-threatening complications of ACS, such as VF, pulseless VT, unstable tachycardias, symptomatic bradycardias, pulmonary edema, cardiogenic shock, and mechanical complications of AMI

Starts "On the Phone" With Activation of EMS

Prompt diagnosis and treatment offers the greatest potential benefit for myocardial salvage. Thus, it is imperative that healthcare providers recognize patients with potential ACS in order to initiate evaluation, appropriate triage, and management as expeditiously as possible.

EMS Components

- Prehospital ECGs
- Notification of the receiving facility of a patient with possible ST-segment elevation myocardial infarction ("STEMI alert")
- Activation of the cardiac catheterization team to shorten reperfusion time
- Continuous review and quality improvement

Hospital-Based Components

- **Emergency department (ED) protocols**
  - Activation of the cardiac catheterization laboratory
  - Admission to the coronary intensive care unit (ICU)
  - Quality assurance, real-time feedback, and healthcare provider education
- **Emergency physician**
  - Empowered to select the most appropriate reperfusion strategy
  - Empowered to activate the cardiac catheterization team as indicated
- **Hospital leadership**
  - Must be involved in the process and committed to support rapid access to STEMI reperfusion therapy

Acute Stroke

The healthcare system has achieved significant improvements in stroke care through integration of public education, emergency dispatch, prehospital detection and triage, hospital stroke system development, and stroke unit management. Not only have the rates of appropriate fibrinolytic therapy increased over the past 5 years, but overall stroke care has also improved, in part through the creation of stroke centers.

Regionalization of Stroke Care

With the National Institute of Neurological Disorders and Stroke (NINDS) recombinant tissue plasminogen activator (rtPA) trial, the crucial need for local partnerships between academic medical centers and community hospitals became clear. The time-sensitive nature of stroke requires such an approach, even in densely populated metropolitan centers.

Community and Professional Education

Community and professional education is essential and has successfully increased the proportion of stroke patients treated with fibrinolytic therapy.

- Patient education efforts are most effective when the message is clear and succinct.
- Educational efforts need to couple the knowledge of the signs and symptoms of stroke with action—activate the emergency response system.

EMS

The integration of EMS into regional stroke models is crucial for improvement of patient outcomes:

- EMS response personnel trained in stroke recognition
- Stroke-prepared hospitals–primary stroke centers
- Access to stroke expertise via telemedicine from the nearest stroke center

Education, Implementation, and Teams

The Chain of Survival is a metaphor used to organize and describe the integrated set of time-sensitive coordinated actions necessary to maximize survival from cardiac arrest. The use of evidence-based education and implementation strategies can optimize the links in the chain.

The Need for Teams

Mortality from in-hospital cardiac arrest remains high. The average survival rate is approximately 21% despite significant advances in treatments. Survival rates are particularly poor for arrest associated with rhythms other than VF/VT. Non-VF/VT rhythms are present in >75% of arrests in the hospital.

Many in-hospital arrests are preceded by easily recognizable physiologic changes, many of which are evident with routine monitoring of vital signs. In recent studies nearly 80% of hospitalized patients with cardiorespiratory arrest had abnormal vital signs documented for up to 8 hours before the actual arrest. This finding suggests that there is a period of increasing instability before the arrest.

Of the small percentage of in-hospital cardiac arrest patients who experience ROSC and are admitted to the ICU, 80% ultimately die before discharge. In comparison, only 44% of nonarrest patients admitted to intensive care urgently from the floor (i.e., before an arrest occurs) die before discharge.

Cardiac Arrest Teams (In-Hospital)

Cardiac arrest teams are unlikely to prevent arrests because their focus has traditionally been to respond only after the arrest has occurred. Unfortunately, the mortality rate is about 80% once the arrest occurs.

Over the past few years, hospitals have shifted the focus away from cardiac arrest teams to patient safety and prevention of arrest. The best way to improve a patient's chance of survival from a cardiorespiratory arrest is to prevent it from happening.

The majority of cardiorespiratory arrests in the hospital should be classified as a "failure to rescue" rather than as an isolated, unexpected, random occurrence. Doing so requires a significant cultural shift within institutions. Actions and interventions need to be proactive with the goal of improving rates of morbidity and mortality rather than reacting to a catastrophic event.

Rapid assessment and intervention for many abnormal physiologic variables can decrease the number of arrests occurring in the hospital.

Rapid Response System

Over the past decade, hospitals in several countries have designed systems to identify and treat early clinical deterioration in patients. The purpose of these rapid response systems is to improve patient outcomes by bringing critical care expertise to patients. The rapid response system has several components:

- Event detection and response triggering arm
- A planned response arm, such as the RRT
- Quality monitoring
- Administrative support

Many rapid response systems allow activation by a nurse, physician, or family member who is concerned that the patient is deteriorating. Some rapid response systems use specific physiologic criteria to determine when to call the team. The following list gives examples of such criteria for adult patients:

- Threatened airway
- Respiratory rate <6 or >30 breaths per minute
- Heart rate <40/min or >140/min
- Systolic blood pressure (SBP) <90 mm Hg
- Symptomatic hypertension
- Unexpected decrease in level of consciousness
- Unexplained agitation
- Seizure
- Significant fall in urine output
- Subjective concern about the patient

Medical Emergency Teams and Rapid Response Teams

There are several names for rapid response systems, including *medical emergency team*, *rapid response team*, and *rapid assessment team*.

The rapid response system is critically dependent on early identification and activation to immediately summon the team to the patient's bedside. These teams typically consist of healthcare providers with both the critical care or emergency care experience and skills to support immediate intervention for life-threatening situations. These teams are responsible for performing a rapid patient assessment and initiating appropriate treatment to reverse physiologic deterioration and prevent a poor outcome.

Regional Systems of Emergency Cardiovascular Care

Hospitals with larger patient volumes have a better survival-to–hospital discharge rate than low-volume centers for patients treated for either in- or out-of-hospital cardiac arrest.

Published Studies

The majority of published "before and after" studies of METs or rapid response systems have reported a 17% to 65% drop in the rate of cardiac arrests after the intervention. Other documented benefits of these systems include:

- A decrease in unplanned emergency transfers to the ICU
- Decreased ICU and total hospital length of stay
- Reductions in postoperative morbidity and mortality rates
- Improved rates of survival from cardiac arrest

The recently published MERIT trial is the only randomized controlled trial comparing hospitals with a MET and those without one. The study did not show a difference in the composite primary outcome (cardiac arrest, unexpected death, unplanned ICU admission) between the 12 hospitals in which a MET system was introduced and 11 hospitals that had no MET system in place. Further research is needed about the critical details of implementation and the potential effectiveness of METs in preventing cardiac arrest or improving other important patient outcomes.

Implementation of a Rapid Response System

Implementing any type of rapid response system will require a significant cultural change in most hospitals. Those who design and manage the system must pay particular attention to issues that may prevent the system from being used effectively. Examples of such issues are insufficient resources, poor education, fear of calling the team, fear of losing control over patient care, and resistance from team members.

Implementation of a rapid response system requires ongoing education, impeccable data collection and review, and feedback. Development and maintenance of these programs requires a long-term cultural and financial commitment from the hospital administration, which must understand that the potential benefits from the system (decreased resource use and improved survival rates) may have independent positive financial ramifications. Hospital administrators and healthcare professionals need to reorient their approach to emergency medical events and develop a culture of patient safety with a primary goal of decreasing morbidity and mortality.

Part 5

The ACLS Cases

Overview of the Cases

The ACLS simulated cases are designed to review the knowledge and skills you need to successfully participate in course events and pass the Megacode skills test. Each case contains the following topics:

- Introduction
- Learning objectives
- Rhythms and drugs
- Descriptions or definitions of key concepts
- Overview of algorithm
- Algorithm figure
- Application of the algorithm to the case
- Other related topics

This part contains the following cases:

Respiratory Arrest Case

Introduction	This case reviews appropriate assessment, intervention, and management options for an *unconscious, unresponsive adult patient in respiratory arrest. Respirations are completely absent or clearly inadequate to maintain effective oxygenation and ventilation. A pulse is present.* (Do not confuse agonal gasps with adequate respirations.) The BLS Survey and the ACLS Survey are used even though the patient is in respiratory arrest and not in cardiac arrest.

Learning Objectives

By the end of this case you should be able to:

1. Describe the use of the BLS and ACLS Surveys for a patient with respiratory arrest with a pulse

2. Describe when airway adjuncts should be used to manage an airway

3. Demonstrate use of an OPA to manage an airway

4. Demonstrate use of an NPA to manage an airway

5. Demonstrate use of bag-mask ventilation to manage an airway

Case Drugs

This case involves the following drugs:

• Oxygen

Systems or facilities using rapid sequence intubation may consider additional drugs.

The BLS Survey

BLS Survey Assessment

Proceed with the BLS Survey Assessment as described on the next page.

Note that the BLS Survey focuses on early CPR and early defibrillation.

IV/IO access is not discussed here even though medications may provide a clinical benefit to some patients. Advanced assessments and interventions are part of the ACLS Survey.

Assess and Reassess the Patient

The systematic approach of the BLS Survey is *assessment,* then *action,* for each step in the sequence.

> ***Remember: Assess...then perform appropriate action.***

In this case you assess and find that the patient has a pulse, so you do not use the AED or begin chest compressions. During the course your instructor will emphasize the need to reassess the patient and be ready to do CPR, attach the AED, and shock the patient if indicated.

Ventilation and Pulse Check

In the case of a patient in respiratory arrest with a pulse, give 1 breath every 5 to 6 seconds (10 to 12 breaths per minute) with a bag-mask or any advanced airway device. Recheck the pulse about every 2 minutes. Take at least 5 seconds but no more than 10 seconds for a pulse check.

	Assess	Assessment Technique and Action	
1	**Check responsive-ness**	• Tap and shout, *"Are you all right?"* • Check for absent or abnormal breathing (no breathing or only gasping) by looking at or **scanning the chest for movement** (about 5 to 10 seconds)	 Check responsiveness.
2	**Activate the emergency response system/get AED**	• Activate the emergency response system and get an AED if one is available or send someone to activate the emergency response system and get an AED or defibrillator	 Activate the emergency response system.

3	**Circulation**	• **Check the carotid pulse** for 5 to 10 seconds
		 • If no pulse within 10 seconds, start CPR (30:2) beginning with chest compressions
		   – Compress the center of the chest (lower half of the sternum) hard and fast with at least 100 compressions per minute at a depth of at least 5 cm (2 inches)
		   – Allow complete chest recoil after each compression
		   – Minimize interruptions in compressions (10 seconds or less)
		   – Switch providers about every 2 minutes to avoid fatigue
		   – Avoid excessive ventilation
		 • If there is a pulse, start rescue breathing at 1 breath every 5 to 6 seconds (10 to 12 breaths per minute). Check pulse about every 2 minutes
			
			 Check the carotid pulse.

4	**Defibrillation**	• If no pulse, check for a shockable rhythm with an AED/defibrillator as soon as it arrives • Provide shocks as indicated • Follow each shock immediately with CPR, beginning with compressions	 Defibrillation.

Ventilation Rates

Airway Device	Ventilations During Cardiac Arrest	Ventilations During Respiratory Arrest
Bag-mask	2 ventilations after every 30 compressions	1 ventilation every 5 to 6 seconds (10 to 12 breaths per minute)
Any advanced airway	1 ventilation every 6 to 8 seconds (8 to 10 breaths per minute)	

The ACLS Survey

Airway Management in Respiratory Arrest

If bag-mask ventilation is adequate, providers may defer insertion of an advanced airway. Healthcare providers should make the decision to place an advanced airway during the ACLS Survey.

Advanced airway equipment includes the laryngeal mask airway, the laryngeal tube, the esophageal-tracheal tube, and the ET tube. If it is within your scope of practice, you may use advanced airway equipment in the course when appropriate and available.

The following is a summary of the ACLS Survey:

Assess	Action as Appropriate

Airway
 	
– *Is the airway patent?*
– *Is an advanced airway indicated?*
– *Is proper placement of airway device confirmed?*
– *Is tube secured and placement reconfirmed frequently?*
	• **Maintain airway patency in unconscious patients** by use of head tilt–chin lift, OPA, or NPA
	• **Use advanced airway management if needed** (e.g., laryngeal mask airway, laryngeal tube, esophageal-tracheal tube, ET tube)
	
	The benefit of advanced airway placement is weighed against the adverse effects of interrupting chest compressions. If bag-mask ventilation is adequate, healthcare providers may defer insertion of an advanced airway until the patient fails to respond to initial CPR and defibrillation or until spontaneous circulation returns. An advanced airway such as a laryngeal mask airway, laryngeal tube, or esophageal-tracheal tube can be placed while chest compressions continue.
	
	If using advanced airway devices:
	
	• **Confirm proper integration of CPR and ventilation**
	• **Confirm proper placement of advanced airway devices** by
	  – Physical examination
	  – Quantitative waveform capnography
	    ■ Class I recommendation for ET tube
	    ■ Reasonable for supraglottic airways
	• **Secure the device to prevent dislodgment**
	• **Monitor airway placement with continuous quantitative waveform capnography**

(continued)

(continued)

Assess	Action as Appropriate

Breathing
 	
– *Are ventilation and oxygenation adequate?*
– *Are quantitative waveform capnography and oxyhemoglobin saturation monitored?*
	• **Give supplementary oxygen when indicated**
	  – For cardiac arrest patients, administer 100% oxygen
	  – For others, titrate oxygen administration to achieve oxygen saturation values of ≥94% by pulse oximetry
	• **Monitor the adequacy of ventilation and oxygenation by**
	  – Clinical criteria (chest rise and cyanosis)
	  – Quantitative waveform capnography
	  – Oxygen saturation
	• **Avoid excessive ventilation**

Circulation
 	
– *What is the cardiac rhythm?*
– *Is the patient with a pulse unstable?*
– *Is defibrillation or cardioversion indicated?*
– *Are chest compressions effective?*
– *Is ROSC present?*
– *Has IV/IO access been established?*
– *Are medications needed for rhythm or blood pressure?*
– *Does the patient need volume (fluid) for resuscitation?*
	• **Monitor CPR quality**
	  – Quantitative waveform capnography (if $P_{ET}CO_2$ is <10 mm Hg, attempt to improve CPR quality)
	  – Intra-arterial pressure (if relaxation phase [diastolic] pressure is <20 mm Hg, attempt to improve CPR quality)
	• **Attach monitor/defibrillator for arrhythmias or cardiac arrest rhythms** (e.g., VF, pulseless VT, asystole, PEA)
	• **Defibrillation/cardioversion**
	• **Obtain IV/IO access**
	• **Give appropriate drugs to manage rhythm and blood pressure**
	• **Give IV/IO fluids if needed**

Differential diagnosis – *Why did this patient develop symptoms or arrest?* – *Is there a reversible cause that can be treated?*	• **Search for, find, and treat reversible causes** (i.e., definitive care)

$P_{ET}CO_2$ is the partial pressure of end-tidal CO_2, a measure of the amount of carbon dioxide present in the exhaled air.

Ventilations

In this case the patient is in respiratory arrest but continues to have a pulse. You should ventilate the patient **once every 5 to 6 seconds** (10 to 12 times per minute). Each breath should take 1 second and achieve visible chest rise. Be careful to avoid excessive ventilation (too many breaths per minute or too large a volume per breath).

FYI 2010 Guidelines **Correct Placement of Endotracheal Tube**	• HSFC recommends continuous waveform capnography in addition to clinical assessment as the most reliable method of confirming and monitoring correct placement of an ET tube.

Management of Respiratory Arrest

Overview

Management of respiratory arrest includes both BLS and ACLS interventions. These interventions may include:

- Giving supplementary oxygen
- Opening the airway
- Providing basic ventilation
- Using basic airway adjuncts (OPA and NPA)
- Suctioning

> *According to the* 2010 Guidelines for CPR and ECC, *for patients with a perfusing rhythm, deliver* 1 breath every 5 to 6 seconds *(10 to 12 breaths per minute).*

Critical Concepts

Avoiding Excessive Ventilation

- When using any form of assisted ventilation, you must avoid delivering excessive ventilation (too many breaths per minute or too large a volume per breath). Excessive ventilation can be harmful because it increases intrathoracic pressure, decreases venous return to the heart, and diminishes cardiac output. It may also cause gastric inflation and predispose the patient to vomiting and aspiration of gastric contents.

Giving Supplementary Oxygen

Maintain Oxygen Saturation

Give oxygen to patients with acute cardiac symptoms or respiratory distress. Monitor oxygen saturation and titrate supplementary oxygen to maintain a saturation of ≥94%.

Opening the Airway

Common Cause of Airway Obstruction

Figure 8 demonstrates the anatomy of the airway. The most common cause of upper airway obstruction in the unconscious/unresponsive patient is loss of tone in the throat muscles. In this case the tongue falls back and occludes the airway at the level of the pharynx (Figure 9A).

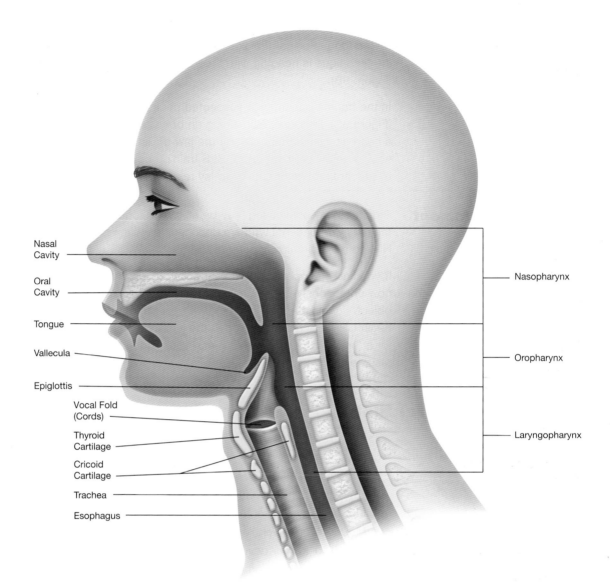

Nasal
Cavity

Oral
Cavity

Tongue

Vallecula

Epiglottis

Vocal Fold
(Cords)

Thyroid
Cartilage

Cricoid
Cartilage

Trachea

Esophagus

Nasopharynx

Oropharynx

Laryngopharynx

Figure 8. Airway anatomy.

A

B

C

Figure 9. Obstruction of the airway by the tongue and epiglottis. When a patient is unresponsive, the tongue can obstruct the airway. The head tilt–chin lift relieves obstruction in the unresponsive patient. **A.** The tongue is obstructing the airway. **B.** The head tilt–chin lift lifts the tongue, relieving the obstruction. **C.** If cervical spine trauma is suspected, healthcare providers should use the jaw thrust without head extension.

Basic Airway Opening Techniques

Basic airway opening techniques will effectively relieve airway obstruction caused either by the tongue or from relaxation of muscles in the upper airway. The basic airway opening technique is head tilt with anterior displacement of the mandible, i.e., head tilt–chin lift (Figure 9B).

In the trauma patient with suspected neck injury, use a jaw thrust without head extension (Figure 9C). Because maintaining an open airway and providing ventilation is a priority, use a head tilt–chin lift maneuver if the jaw thrust does not open the airway. ACLS providers should be aware that current BLS training courses teach the jaw thrust technique to healthcare providers but not to lay rescuers.

Airway Management

Proper airway positioning may be all that is required for patients who can breathe spontaneously. In patients who are unconscious with no cough or gag reflex, insert an OPA or NPA to maintain airway patency.

If you find an unconscious/unresponsive patient who was known to be choking and is now unresponsive and in respiratory arrest, open the mouth wide and look for a foreign object. If you see one, remove it with your fingers. If you do not see a foreign object, begin CPR. Each time you open the airway to give breaths, open the mouth wide and look for a foreign object. Remove it with your fingers if present. If there is no foreign object, resume CPR.

Providing Basic Ventilation

Basic Airway Skills

Basic airway skills used to ventilate a patient are:

- Head tilt–chin lift
- Jaw thrust without head extension (suspected cervical spine trauma)
- Mouth-to-mouth ventilation
- Mouth-to-nose ventilation
- Mouth-to–barrier device (using a pocket mask) ventilation (Figure 10)
- Bag-mask ventilation (Figures 11 and 12)

Figure 10. Mouth-to-mask ventilation, 1 rescuer. The rescuer performs 1-rescuer CPR from a position at the patient's side. Perform a head tilt–chin lift to open the airway while holding the mask tightly against the face.

Figure 11. E-C clamp technique for holding the mask while lifting the jaw. Position yourself at the patient's head. Circle the thumb and first finger around the top of the mask (forming a "C") while using the third, fourth, and fifth fingers (forming an "E") to lift the jaw.

Figure 12. Two-rescuer use of the bag-mask. The rescuer at the patient's head tilts the patient's head and seals the mask against the patient's face with the thumb and first finger of each hand creating a "C" to provide a complete seal around the edges of the mask. The rescuer uses the remaining 3 fingers (the "E") to lift the jaw (this holds the airway open). The second rescuer slowly squeezes the bag (over 1 second) until the chest rises. Both providers should observe chest rise.

Bag-Mask Ventilation

A bag-mask ventilation device consists of a ventilation bag attached to a face mask. These devices have been a mainstay of emergency ventilation for decades. Bag-mask devices are the most common method of providing positive-pressure ventilation. When using a bag-mask device, deliver approximately 600 mL tidal volume sufficient to produce chest rise over 1 second.

The universal connections present on all airway devices allow you to connect any ventilation bag to numerous adjuncts. Valves and ports may include:

- One-way valves to prevent the patient from rebreathing exhaled air
- Oxygen ports for administering supplementary oxygen
- Medication ports for administering aerosolized and other medications
- Suction ports for clearing the airway
- Ports for quantitative sampling of end-tidal CO_2

You can attach other adjuncts to the patient end of the valve, including a pocket face mask, laryngeal mask airway, laryngeal tube, esophageal-tracheal tube, and ET tube.

Basic Airway Adjuncts: Oropharyngeal Airway

Introduction

The OPA is used in patients who are at risk for developing airway obstruction from the tongue or from relaxed upper airway muscles. This J-shaped device (Figure 13A) fits over the tongue to hold it and the soft hypopharyngeal structures away from the posterior wall of the pharynx.

The OPA is used in *unconscious* patients if procedures to open the airway (e.g., head tilt–chin lift or jaw thrust) fail to provide and maintain a clear, unobstructed airway. *An OPA should not be used in a conscious or semiconscious patient* because it may stimulate gagging and vomiting. The key assessment is to check whether the patient has an intact cough and gag reflex. If so, do not use an OPA.

The OPA may be used to keep the airway open during bag-mask ventilation when providers might unknowingly push down on the chin, blocking the airway. The OPA is also used during suctioning of the mouth and throat and in intubated patients to prevent them from biting and occluding the ET tube.

A **B**

Figure 13. Oropharyngeal airways. **A.** Oropharyngeal airway devices. **B.** Oropharyngeal airway device inserted.

Technique of OPA Insertion

Step	Action
1	**Clear the mouth and pharynx** of secretions, blood, or vomit using a rigid pharyngeal suction tip if possible.
2	**Select the proper size OPA.** Place the OPA against the side of the face. When the tip of the OPA is at the corner of the mouth, the flange is at the angle of the mandible. A properly sized and inserted OPA results in proper alignment with the glottic opening.
3	**Insert the OPA** so that it curves upward toward the hard palate as it enters the mouth.
4	As the OPA passes through the oral cavity and approaches the posterior wall of the pharynx, **rotate it 180°** into the proper position (Figure 13B). The OPA can also be inserted at a 90° angle to the mouth and then turned down toward the posterior pharynx as it is advanced. In both methods, the goal is to curve the device around the tongue so that the tongue is not inadvertently pushed back into the pharynx rather than being pulled forward by the OPA. An **alternative method** is to insert the OPA straight in while using a tongue depressor or similar device to hold the tongue forward as the OPA is advanced.

After insertion of an OPA, monitor the patient. Keep the head and jaw positioned properly to maintain a patent airway. Suction the airway as needed.

Caution

Be Aware of the Following When Using an OPA

- OPAs that are *too large* may obstruct the larynx or cause trauma to the laryngeal structures.
- OPAs that are *too small* or inserted improperly may push the base of the tongue posteriorly and obstruct the airway.
- Insert the OPA carefully to avoid soft tissue trauma to the lips and tongue.

Remember to use the OPA only in the unresponsive patient with *no cough or gag reflex*. If the patient has a cough or gag reflex, the OPA may stimulate vomiting and laryngospasm.

Basic Airway Adjuncts: Nasopharyngeal Airway

Introduction

The NPA is used as an alternative to an OPA in patients who need a basic airway management adjunct. The NPA is a soft rubber or plastic uncuffed tube (Figure 14A) that provides a conduit for airflow between the nares and the pharynx.

Unlike oral airways, NPAs *may be used in conscious or semiconscious patients* (patients with an intact cough and gag reflex). The NPA is indicated when insertion of an OPA is technically difficult or dangerous. Examples include patients with a gag reflex, trismus, massive trauma around the mouth, or wiring of the jaws. The NPA may also be used in patients who are neurologically impaired with poor pharyngeal tone or coordination leading to upper airway obstruction.

A   B

Figure 14. Nasopharyngeal airways. **A.** Nasopharyngeal airway devices. **B.** Nasopharyngeal airway device inserted.

Technique of NPA Insertion

Step	Action
1	**Select the proper size NPA.** • Compare the outer circumference of the NPA with the inner aperture of the nares. The NPA should not be so large that it causes sustained blanching of the nostrils. Some providers use the diameter of the patient's smallest finger as a guide to selecting the proper size. • The length of the NPA should be the same as the distance from the tip of the patient's nose to the earlobe.
2	**Lubricate the airway with a water-soluble lubricant or anesthetic jelly.**
3	**Insert the airway** through the nostril in a posterior direction perpendicular to the plane of the face. Pass it gently along the floor of the nasopharynx (Figure 14B). If you encounter resistance: • Slightly rotate the tube to facilitate insertion at the angle of the nasal passage and nasopharynx. • Attempt placement through the other nostril because patients have different-sized nasal passages.

Reevaluate frequently. Maintain head tilt by providing anterior displacement of the mandible using a chin lift or jaw thrust. Mucus, blood, vomit, or the soft tissues of the pharynx can obstruct the NPA, which has a small internal diameter. *Frequent evaluation and suctioning of the airway may be necessary to ensure patency.*

Caution **Be Aware of the Following When Using an NPA**	• Take care to insert the airway gently to avoid complications. The airway can irritate the mucosa or lacerate adenoidal tissue and cause bleeding, with possible aspiration of clots into the trachea. Suction may be necessary to remove blood or secretions. • An improperly sized NPA may enter the esophagus. With active ventilation, such as bag-mask ventilation, the NPA may cause gastric inflation and possible hypoventilation. • An NPA may cause laryngospasm and vomiting, even though it is commonly tolerated by semiconscious patients. • Use caution in patients with facial trauma because of the risk of misplacement into the cranial cavity through a fractured cribriform plate.

Foundational Facts **Precautions for OPAs and NPAs**	Take the following precautions when using an OPA or NPA: • Always check spontaneous respirations immediately after insertion of either an OPA or an NPA. • If respirations are absent or inadequate, start positive-pressure ventilations at once with an appropriate device. • If adjuncts are unavailable, use mouth-to-mask barrier device ventilation.

Suctioning

Introduction

Suctioning is an essential component of maintaining a patient's airway. Providers should suction the airway immediately if there are copious secretions, blood, or vomit.

Suction devices consist of both portable and wall-mounted units.

- Portable suction devices are easy to transport but may not provide adequate suction power. A suction force of −80 to −120 mm Hg is generally necessary.
- Wall-mounted suction units should be capable of providing an airflow of >40 L/min at the end of the delivery tube and a vacuum of more than −300 mm Hg when the tube is clamped at full suction.
- Adjust the amount of suction force for use in children and intubated patients.

Soft vs Rigid Catheters

Both soft flexible and rigid suctioning catheters are available.

Soft flexible catheters may be used in the mouth or nose. Soft flexible catheters are available in sterile wrappers and can also be used for ET tube deep suctioning.

Rigid catheters (e.g., Yankauer) are used to suction the oropharynx. These are better for suctioning thick secretions and particulate matter.

Catheter Type	Use for
Soft	• Aspiration of thin secretions from the oropharynx and nasopharynx • Performing intratracheal suctioning • Suctioning through an in-place airway (i.e., NPA) to access the back of the pharynx in a patient with clenched teeth
Rigid	• More effective suctioning of the oropharynx, particularly if there is thick particulate matter

Oropharyngeal Suctioning Procedure

Follow the steps below to perform oropharyngeal suctioning.

Step	Action
1	• Measure the catheter before suctioning and do not insert it any further than the distance from the tip of the nose to the earlobe. • Gently insert the suction catheter or device into the oropharynx beyond the tongue.
2	• Apply suction by occluding the side opening of the catheter while withdrawing with a rotating or twisting motion. • If using a rigid suction device (e.g., Yankauer suction) place the tip gently into the oral cavity. Advance by pushing the tongue down to reach the oropharynx if necessary.

Endotracheal Tube Suctioning Procedure

Patients with pulmonary secretions may require suctioning even after endotracheal intubation. Follow the steps below to perform ET tube suctioning:

Step	Action
1	• Use sterile technique to reduce the likelihood of airway contamination.
2	• Gently insert the catheter into the ET tube. Be sure the side opening is not occluded during insertion. Insertion of the catheter beyond the tip of the ET tube is not recommended because it may injure the endotracheal mucosa or stimulate coughing or bronchospasm.
3	• Apply suction by occluding the side opening only while withdrawing the catheter with a rotating or twisting motion. • **Suction attempts should not exceed 10 seconds.** To avoid hypoxemia, precede and follow suctioning attempts with a short period of administration of 100% oxygen.

> *Monitor the patient's heart rate, pulse, oxygen saturation, and clinical appearance during suctioning. If bradycardia develops, oxygen saturation drops, or clinical appearance deteriorates, interrupt suctioning at once. Administer high-flow oxygen until the heart rate returns to normal and the clinical condition improves. Assist ventilation as needed.*

Providing Ventilation With an Advanced Airway

Introduction

Selection of an advanced airway device depends on the training, scope of practice, and equipment of the providers on the resuscitation team. Advanced airways include:

- Laryngeal mask airway
- Laryngeal tube
- Esophageal-tracheal tube
- Endotracheal tube

Because a small proportion of patients cannot be ventilated with a laryngeal mask airway, providers who use this device should have an alternative airway management strategy. A bag-mask can be this alternate strategy.

This course will familiarize you with types of advanced airways. Instruction in the skilled placement of these airways is beyond the scope of the basic ACLS Provider Course. To be proficient in the use of advanced airway devices, you must have adequate initial training and ongoing experience. Providers who insert advanced airways must participate in a process of continuous quality improvement to document and minimize complications.

In this course you will practice ventilating with an advanced airway in place and integrating ventilation with chest compressions.

Ventilation Rates

Airway Device	Ventilations During Cardiac Arrest	Ventilations During Respiratory Arrest
Bag-mask	2 ventilations after every 30 compressions	**1 ventilation every 5 to 6 seconds** (10 to 12 breaths per minute)
Any advanced airway	**1 ventilation every 6 to 8 seconds** (8 to 10 breaths per minute)	

Laryngeal Mask Airway

The laryngeal mask airway is an advanced airway alternative to endotracheal intubation and provides comparable ventilation. It is acceptable to use the laryngeal mask airway as an alternative to an ET tube for airway management in cardiac arrest. Only experienced providers should perform laryngeal mask airway insertion.

Laryngeal Tube

The advantages of the laryngeal tube are similar to those of the esophageal-tracheal tube; however, the laryngeal tube is more compact and less complicated to insert.

Healthcare professionals trained in the use of the laryngeal tube may consider it as an alternative to bag-mask ventilation or endotracheal intubation for airway management in cardiac arrest. Only experienced providers should perform laryngeal tube insertion.

Esophageal-Tracheal Tube

The esophageal-tracheal tube is an advanced airway alternative to endotracheal intubation. This device provides adequate ventilation comparable to an ET tube. It is acceptable to use the esophageal-tracheal tube as an alternative to an ET tube for airway management in cardiac arrest. Fatal complications may occur with use of this device. Only providers experienced with its use should perform esophageal-tracheal tube insertion.

Endotracheal Tube

A brief summary of the basic steps for performing endotracheal intubation is given here to familiarize the ACLS provider who may assist with the procedure.

- Prepare for intubation by assembling the necessary equipment.
- Perform endotracheal intubation.
- Inflate cuff or cuffs on the tube.
- Attach the ventilation bag.
- Confirm correct placement by physical examination and a confirmation device. Continuous waveform capnography is recommended (in addition to clinical assessment) as the most reliable method of confirming and monitoring correct placement of an ET tube. Healthcare providers may use colorimetric and nonwaveform carbon dioxide detectors when waveform capnography is not available.
- Secure the tube in place.
- Monitor for displacement.

Only experienced providers should perform endotracheal intubation.

Caution
Use of Cricoid Pressure

- Cricoid pressure in nonarrest patients may offer some measure of protection to the airway from aspiration and gastric insufflation during bag-mask ventilation. However, it also may impede ventilation and interfere with placement of a supraglottic airway or intubation.

FYI 2010 Guidelines
Cricoid Pressure

- The role of cricoid pressure during out-of-hospital and in-hospital cardiac arrest has not been studied. If cricoid pressure is used in a few special circumstances during cardiac arrest, the pressure should be adjusted, relaxed, or released if it impedes ventilation or advanced airway placement. The routine use of cricoid pressure in cardiac arrest is not recommended.

Foundational Facts
Rescue Breaths for CPR With an Advanced Airway in Place

- During CPR the compression-to-ventilation ratio is 30:2. But once an advanced airway is in place (i.e., laryngeal mask airway, laryngeal tube, esophageal-tracheal tube, or ET tube), chest compressions are no longer interrupted for ventilations.
- When ventilating through a properly placed advanced airway, give 1 breath every 6 to 8 seconds (approximately 8 to 10 breaths per minute) without trying to synchronize breaths to compressions. Ideally deliver the breath during chest recoil between compressions. Continuously reevaluate compressions and ventilations. Be prepared to make modifications if either is ineffective.

In this case the patient has a pulse, and compressions are not indicated. Give 1 breath every 5 to 6 seconds (10 to 12 breaths per minute).

Precautions for Trauma Patients

Summary

When providing assisted ventilation for patients with known or suspected cervical spine trauma, avoid unnecessary spine movement. Excessive head and neck movement in patients with an unstable cervical spinal column can cause irreversible injury to the spinal cord or worsen a minor spinal cord injury. Approximately 2% of patients with blunt trauma serious enough to require spinal imaging in the ED have a spinal injury. This risk is tripled if the patient has a head or facial injury. Assume that any patient with multiple trauma, head injury, or facial trauma has a spine injury. Be particularly cautious if a patient has suspected cervical spine injury. Examples are patients who have been involved in a high-speed motor vehicle collision, have fallen from a height, or were injured while diving.

Follow these precautions if you suspect cervical spine trauma:

- Open the airway by using a jaw thrust *without head extension*. Because maintaining a patent airway and providing adequate ventilation are priorities, use a head tilt–chin lift maneuver if the jaw thrust is not effective.
- Have another team member stabilize the head in a neutral position during airway manipulation. *Use manual spinal motion restriction rather than immobilization devices.* Manual spinal immobilization is safer. Cervical collars may complicate airway management and may even interfere with airway patency.
- Spinal immobilization devices are helpful during transport.

VF Treated With CPR and AED Case

Introduction

This case will provide the knowledge you need to pass the CPR and AED Testing Station. This case discusses how to respond as a lone rescuer to an out-of-hospital emergency, equipped with only CPR skills and an AED. The case scenario presents a *patient who collapses from either VF or pulseless VT*. The only equipment available is an AED stocked with a pocket face mask. Because other providers are not present, you must care for the patient without help.

ACLS interventions, including advanced airway control and IV medications, are not options in this scenario.

Note that during the course you will be required to demonstrate both your knowledge of this case and competency in basic skill performance.

Learning Objectives

By the end of this case you should be able to:

1. Demonstrate the skills and sequence outlined in the BLS Healthcare Providers Algorithm (Figures 15 and 16), including high-quality CPR and AED use

2. Implement the BLS Healthcare Provider Algorithm by performing 1-rescuer CPR

3. Implement the BLS Healthcare Provider Algorithm by operating an AED

Rhythms for VF Treated With CPR and AED

With an AED, there are no rhythms to learn. The AED will answer the question "Is the rhythm shockable, i.e., VF or pulseless VT?"

Drugs for VF Treated With CPR and AED

There are no new drugs to learn in this case. You will use only your CPR skills and an AED.

The BLS Survey

Introduction

The BLS Survey is used in all cases of cardiac arrest.

In the Respiratory Arrest Case you learned the basics of airway assessment and management of a patient in respiratory arrest with a pulse. In this case you will assess and manage a patient without a pulse and use the AED.

Assessment

Perform the BLS Survey steps on the next page.

Foundational Facts **Starting CPR When You Are Not Sure About a Pulse**	• If you are unsure about the presence of a pulse, begin cycles of compressions and ventilations. Unnecessary compressions are less harmful than failing to provide compressions when needed. Delaying or failing to start CPR in a patient without a pulse reduces the chance of survival.

	Assess	Assessment Technique and Action	
1	**Check responsiveness**	• Tap and shout, ***"Are you all right?"*** • Check for absent or abnormal breathing (no breathing or only gasping) by looking at or **scanning the chest for movement** (about 5 to 10 seconds)	 Check responsiveness.
2	**Activate the emergency response system/get AED**	• Activate the emergency response system and get an AED if one is available or send someone to activate the emergency response system and get an AED or defibrillator	 Activate the emergency response system.

3	**Circulation**	• **Check the carotid pulse** for 5 to 10 seconds
		• If no pulse within 10 seconds, start CPR (30:2) beginning with chest compressions
		  – Compress the center of the chest (lower half of the sternum) hard and fast with at least 100 compressions per minute at a depth of at least 5 cm (2 inches)
		  – Allow complete chest recoil after each compression
		  – Minimize interruptions in compressions (10 seconds or less)
		  – Switch providers about every 2 minutes to avoid fatigue
		  – Avoid excessive ventilation
		• If there is a pulse, start rescue breathing at 1 breath every 5 to 6 seconds (10 to 12 breaths per minute). Check pulse about every 2 minutes
			
			Check the carotid pulse.

4	**Defibrillation**	• If no pulse, check for a shockable rhythm with an AED/defibrillator as soon as it arrives • Provide shocks as indicated • Follow each shock immediately with CPR, beginning with compressions	 Defibrillation.

Adult BLS Healthcare Providers

1 | Unresponsive
No breathing or no normal breathing
(i.e., only gasping)

2 | Activate emergency response system
Get AED/defibrillator
or send second rescuer (if available) to do this

High-Quality CPR
- Rate at least 100/min
- Compression depth at least 5 cm (2 inches)
- Allow complete chest recoil after each compression
- Minimize interruptions in chest compressions
- Avoid excessive ventilation

3 | Check pulse:
DEFINITE pulse
within 10 seconds?

Definite Pulse →

3A |
- Give 1 breath every 5 to 6 seconds
- Recheck pulse every 2 minutes

No Pulse

4 | Begin cycles of **30 COMPRESSIONS** and **2 BREATHS**

5 | AED/defibrillator ARRIVES

6 | Check rhythm
Shockable rhythm?

Shockable

Not Shockable

7 | Give 1 shock
Resume CPR immediately
for 2 minutes

8 | Resume CPR immediately
for 2 minutes
Check rhythm every
2 minutes; continue until
ALS providers take over or
victim starts to move

Note: The boxes bordered with dashed lines are performed by healthcare providers and not by lay rescuers

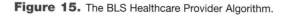

Figure 15. The BLS Healthcare Provider Algorithm.

Simplified Adult BLS HCP

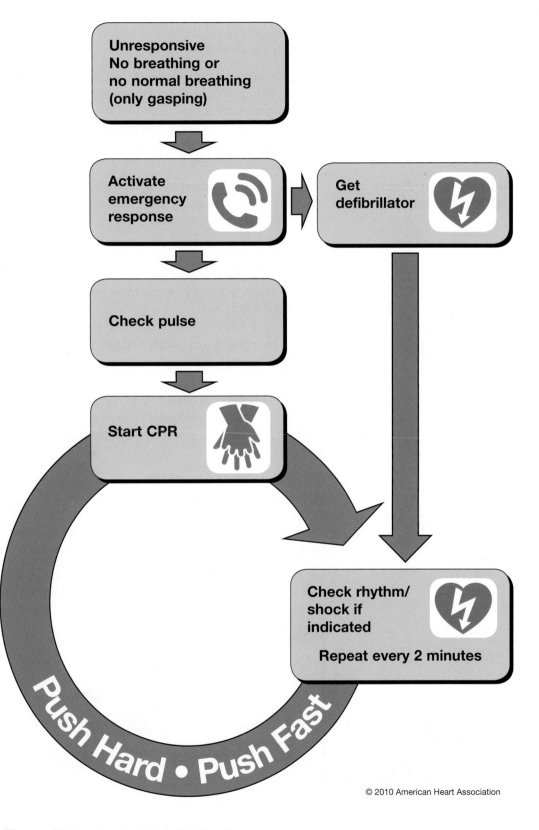

Figure 16. The Simplified Adult BLS Algorithm.

Purpose of Defibrillation

Defibrillation does not restart the heart. Defibrillation stuns the heart and briefly terminates all electrical activity, including VF and VT. If the heart is still viable, its normal pacemakers may eventually resume electrical activity (return of spontaneous rhythm) that ultimately results in a perfusing rhythm (ROSC).

In the first minutes after successful defibrillation, however, any spontaneous rhythm is typically slow and does not create pulses or adequate perfusion. The patient needs CPR (beginning with chest compressions) for several minutes until adequate heart function resumes. This is the rationale for resuming high-quality CPR, beginning with chest compressions immediately after a shock.

Principle of Early Defibrillation

The interval from collapse to defibrillation is one of the most important determinants of survival from cardiac arrest. Early defibrillation is critical for patients with sudden cardiac arrest for the following reasons:

- A common initial rhythm in out-of-hospital witnessed sudden cardiac arrest is VF. Pulseless VT rapidly deteriorates to VF. When VF is present, the heart quivers and does not pump blood.
- Electrical defibrillation is the most effective way to treat VF (delivery of a shock to stop the VF).
- The probability of successful defibrillation decreases quickly over time.
- VF deteriorates to asystole if not treated.

The earlier defibrillation occurs, the higher the survival rate. When VF is present, CPR can provide a small amount of blood flow to the heart and brain but cannot directly restore an organized rhythm. The likelihood of restoring a perfusing rhythm is optimized with immediate CPR and defibrilliation within a few minutes of the initial arrest. Restoration of a perfusing rhythm requires immediate CPR and defibrillation within a few minutes of the initial arrest (Figure 17).

For every minute that passes between collapse and defibrillation, the chance of survival from a witnessed VF sudden cardiac arrest declines by 7% to 10% per minute if no bystander CPR is provided. When bystanders perform CPR, the decline is more gradual and averages 3% to 4% per minute. CPR performed early can double or triple survival from witnessed sudden cardiac arrest at most defibrillation intervals.

Lay rescuer AED programs increase the likelihood of early CPR and attempted defibrillation. This helps shorten the time between collapse and defibrillation for a greater number of patients with sudden cardiac arrest.

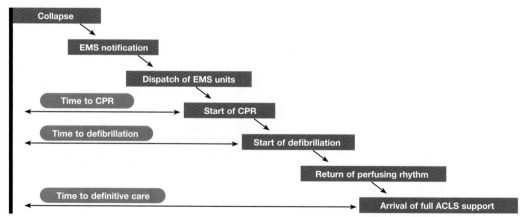

Figure 17. Sequence of events and key intervals that occur with cardiac arrest.

Modified from Eisenberg MS, Cummins RO, Damon S, Larsen MP, Hearne TR. Survival rates from out-of-hospital cardiac arrest: recommendations for uniform definitions and data to report. *Ann Emerg Med.* 1990;19:1249-1259. With permission from Elsevier.

AED Operation

Use AEDs only when patients have the following 3 clinical findings:

- No response
- Absent or abnormal breathing (i.e., no breathing or only gasping)
- No pulse

In the first few minutes after the onset of sudden cardiac arrest, the patient may demonstrate agonal gasps, which are *not* adequate breathing. A nonresponsive patient with agonal gasping who has no pulse is in cardiac arrest.

Critical Concepts Agonal Gasps	**Agonal gasps are not adequate breathing.** A patient who gasps usually looks like he is drawing air in very quickly. The patient may open his mouth and move his jaw, head, or neck. Gasps may appear forceful or weak, and some time may pass between gasps because they usually happen at a slow rate. The gasp may sound like a snort, snore, or groan. Gasping is not regular or normal breathing. It is a sign of cardiac arrest in someone who doesn't respond.

Know Your AED

You must be familiar with the AED used in your clinical setting and be ready to use it at any time. Review the troubleshooting checklist supplied by the AED manufacturer. Learn to perform daily maintenance checks. Not only are these checks an effective review of the steps of operation, but they are also a means of verifying that the AED is ready for use.

The Universal AED: Common Steps to Operate All AEDs

Once the AED arrives, place it at the patient's side, next to the rescuer who will operate it. This position provides ready access to the AED controls and easy placement of electrode pads. It also allows a second rescuer to perform CPR from the opposite side of the patient without interfering with AED operation.

AEDs are available in different models. Although there are small differences from model to model, all AEDs operate in basically the same way. The following table lists the 4 universal steps for operating an AED:

Step	Action
1	**Power on the AED** (this activates voice prompts for guidance in all subsequent steps). • Open the carrying case or the top of the AED. • Turn the power on (some devices will "power on" automatically when you open the lid or case).

2	**Attach electrode pads** to the patient's bare chest.
	
	• Choose the correct size pads (adult versus pediatric) for the patient's size/age. Peel the backing away from the electrode pads.
	• Quickly wipe the patient's chest if it is covered with water or sweat (but do not delay attaching the pads or shock delivery).
	• Attach the adhesive electrode pads to the patient's bare chest.
	  – Place one electrode pad on the upper-right side of the bare chest to the right of the sternum directly below the clavicle.
	  – Place the other pad to the left of the nipple, with the top margin of the pad about 5 cm below the left armpit (Figure 18).
	  – Attach the AED connecting cables to the AED box (some are preconnected).

(continued)

(continued)

Step	Action
3	**Analyze rhythm.** • Always clear the patient during analysis. Be sure no one is touching the patient, not even the person in charge of giving breaths. • Some AEDs will instruct you to push a button to allow the AED to begin analyzing the heart rhythm; others will do that automatically. The AED rhythm analysis may take about 5 to 15 seconds. • The AED rhythm analysis will determine if the patient needs a shock.
4	If the AED advises a shock, it will tell you to **BE SURE TO CLEAR THE PATIENT (i.e., do not touch the patient):** • Clear the patient before delivering the shock; be sure no one is touching the patient. • Loudly and quickly state a "clear the patient" message, such as "Clear, I am going to shock on three," "One, two, three, shocking," or simply "Clear." • Perform a visual check to ensure that no one is in contact with the patient. • Press the **SHOCK** button. • The shock will produce a sudden contraction of the patient's muscles.

As soon as the shock is delivered, resume CPR, starting with chest compressions, and give cycles of 30 compressions and 2 breaths. Do not perform a pulse or rhythm check. After 2 minutes of CPR the AED will prompt you to repeat steps 3 and 4.

Figure 18. AED electrode pad placement on the patient.

Foundational Facts **Alternative AED Electrode Pad Placement Positions**	There are 4 acceptable AED electrode pad positions: • Anterolateral • Anteroposterior • Anterior-left infrascapular • Anterior-right infrascapular All 4 positions are equally effective in shock success and are reasonable for defibrillation. For ease of placement, anterolateral is a reasonable default electrode placement. Providers may consider alternative pad positions based on individual patient characteristics.

Troubleshooting the AED	Studies of AED "failures" have shown that most problems are caused by operator error rather than by AED defects. Operator error is less likely if the operator is experienced in using the AED, has had recent training or practice with the AED, and is using a well-maintained AED. If the AED does not promptly analyze the rhythm, do the following: • Resume high-quality chest compressions and ventilations. • Check all connections between the AED and the patient to make sure that they are intact. *Never delay chest compressions to troubleshoot the AED.*

Shock First vs CPR First	When you care for an adult patient in cardiac arrest, should you attempt to shock first with an AED or provide CPR first? • Healthcare providers who treat cardiac arrest in hospitals and other facilities should provide immediate CPR until the AED/defibrillator is ready for use. Use the AED as soon as it is available. • At this time the benefit of delaying defibrillation to perform CPR before defibrillation is unclear. EMS system medical directors may consider implementing a protocol that allows EMS responders to provide CPR while preparing for defibrillation of patients found by EMS personnel to be in VF.

FYI 2010 Guidelines **Coordinating Shock Delivery and CPR**	• HSFC strongly recommends performing CPR while a defibrillator or AED is readied for use and while charging for all patients in cardiac arrest. • Responders using an AED should follow the machine's voice prompts.

AED Use in Special Situations

Introduction	The following special situations may require the operator to take extra care in placing the electrode pads when using an AED.

Hairy Chest	If the patient has a hairy chest, the AED pads may stick to the hair and not to the skin on the chest. If this occurs, the AED will not properly analyze the patient's heart rhythm. The AED will give a "check electrodes" or "check electrode pads" message. If this happens, complete the following steps and actions while minimizing interruptions in chest compressions.

Part 5

Step	Action
1	If the pads stick to the hair instead of the skin, press down firmly on each pad.
2	If the AED continues to prompt you to "check pads" or "check electrodes," quickly pull off the pads. This will remove much of the hair.
3	If too much hair remains where you will put the pads, shave the area with the razor in the AED carrying case, if available.
4	Put on a new set of pads. Follow the AED voice prompts.

Water

Do not use an AED in the water.

If water is present on the patient's chest, it may conduct the shock electricity across the skin of the chest. This will prevent the delivery of an adequate shock dose to the heart.

If...	Then...
The patient is in the water	Pull the patient out of the water
The patient's chest is covered with water	Wipe the chest quickly before attaching the electrodes
The patient is lying on snow or ice or in a small puddle	Use the AED

Implanted Pacemaker

Patients known to be at high risk for sudden cardiac arrest may have implanted defibrillators/pacemakers that automatically deliver shocks directly to the heart muscle if a life-threatening arrhythmia is detected. You can immediately identify these devices because they create a hard lump beneath the skin of the upper chest or abdomen. The lump ranges in size from the size of a silver dollar to half the size of a deck of cards, with a small overlying scar. The presence of an implanted defibrillator or pacemaker is not a contraindication to attaching and using an AED. Avoid placing the AED electrode pads directly over the device because the devices may interfere with each other.

If you identify an implanted defibrillator/pacemaker:

- If possible, place the AED electrode pad to either side and not directly on top of the implanted device.
- Follow the normal steps for operating an AED.

Occasionally the analysis and shock cycles of implanted defibrillators and AEDs will conflict. If the implanted defibrillator is delivering shocks to the patient (the patient's muscles contract in a manner like that observed after an AED shock), allow 30 to 60 seconds for the implanted defibrillator to complete the treatment cycle before delivering a shock from the AED.

Transdermal Medication Patches

Do not place AED electrodes directly on top of a medication patch (e.g., a patch of nitroglycerin, nicotine, pain medication, hormone replacement therapy, or antihypertensive medication). The medication patch may block the transfer of energy from the electrode pad to the heart or cause small burns to the skin. To prevent these complications, remove the patch and wipe the area clean before attaching the AED electrode pad. Try to minimize interruptions in chest compressions and do not delay shock delivery.

VF/Pulseless VT Case

Introduction

This case focuses on the assessment and actions used for a witnessed cardiac arrest due to VF or pulseless VT that is refractory (unresponsive) to the first shock. You will use a manual defibrillator in this case.

In this case and during the course you will have an opportunity to demonstrate effective resuscitation team behaviors while performing the assessment and action skills. During the BLS Survey, team members will perform continuous high-quality CPR with effective chest compressions and ventilation with a bag-mask device. The team leader will conduct the ACLS Survey, including rhythm recognition (shockable versus nonshockable), defibrillation using a manual defibrillator, resuscitation drugs, a discussion of IV/IO access, and advanced airways.

The success of any resuscitation attempt is built on a strong base of high-quality CPR and defibrillation when required by the patient's ECG rhythm.

Learning Objectives

By the end of this case you should be able to:

1. Describe signs that the patient is experiencing VF/pulseless VT

2. Recognize VF and VT on the ECG

3. Manage VF/pulseless VT according to the Cardiac Arrest Algorithm

4. Recall indications for drugs recommended for refractory VF/pulseless VT

5. Recall contraindications for drugs recommended for refractory VF/pulseless VT

6. Recall doses for drugs recommended for refractory VF/pulseless VT

7. Recall routes of administration for drugs recommended for refractory VF/pulseless VT

8. State appropriate electrical doses used for VF/pulseless VT arrest

9. Perform defibrillation with minimal (10 seconds or less) interruption of chest compressions

10. ROSC: Support blood pressure with fluids

11. ROSC: Support blood pressure with pressors

12. ROSC: Ensure ventilation by using quantitative waveform capnography

13. ROSC: Titrate FIO_2 by using pulse oximetry

14. ROSC: Assess for STEMI: 12-lead and intervention

15. ROSC: Assess level of consciousness

16. ROSC: Consider hypothermia for comatose patients

17. ROSC: Treat reversible causes

18. ROSC: Place patient into appropriate system of care

Rhythms for VF/ Pulseless VT

This case involves these ECG rhythms:

- VF
- VT
- ECG artifact that looks like VF
- New left bundle branch block

Drugs for VF/ Pulseless VT

This case involves these drugs:

- Epinephrine
- Norepinephrine
- Vasopressin
- Amiodarone
- Lidocaine
- Magnesium sulfate
- Dopamine
- Oxygen

Managing VF/Pulseless VT: The Cardiac Arrest Algorithm

Overview

The Cardiac Arrest Algorithm (Figure 19) is the most important algorithm to know for adult resuscitation. This algorithm outlines all assessment and management steps for the pulseless patient who does not initially respond to BLS interventions, including a first shock from an AED. The 2005 algorithm was simplified and redesigned to emphasize the importance of minimally interrupted high-quality CPR. The algorithm consists of the 2 pathways for a cardiac arrest:

- A shockable rhythm (VF/pulseless VT) displayed on the left side of the algorithm
- A nonshockable rhythm (asystole/PEA) displayed on the right side of the algorithm

Throughout the case discussion of the Cardiac Arrest Algorithm, we will refer to Boxes 1 through 12. These are the numbers assigned to the boxes on the algorithm.

VF/VT (Left Side)

Because many patients with sudden cardiac arrest demonstrate VF at some point in their arrest, it is likely that ACLS providers will frequently follow the left side of the Cardiac Arrest Algorithm (Figure 19). Rapid treatment of VF according to this sequence is the best scientific approach to restoring spontaneous circulation.

Pulseless VT is included in the algorithm because it is treated as VF. VF and pulseless VT require CPR until a defibrillator is available. Both are treated with high-energy unsynchronized shocks.

Asystole/PEA (Right Side)

The right side of the algorithm outlines the sequence of actions to perform if the rhythm is nonshockable. You will have an opportunity to practice this sequence in the asystole and PEA cases.

Summary

The VF/Pulseless VT Case gives you the opportunity to practice performing rapid treatment of VF/VT by following the steps on the left side of the Cardiac Arrest Algorithm (Boxes 1 through 8).

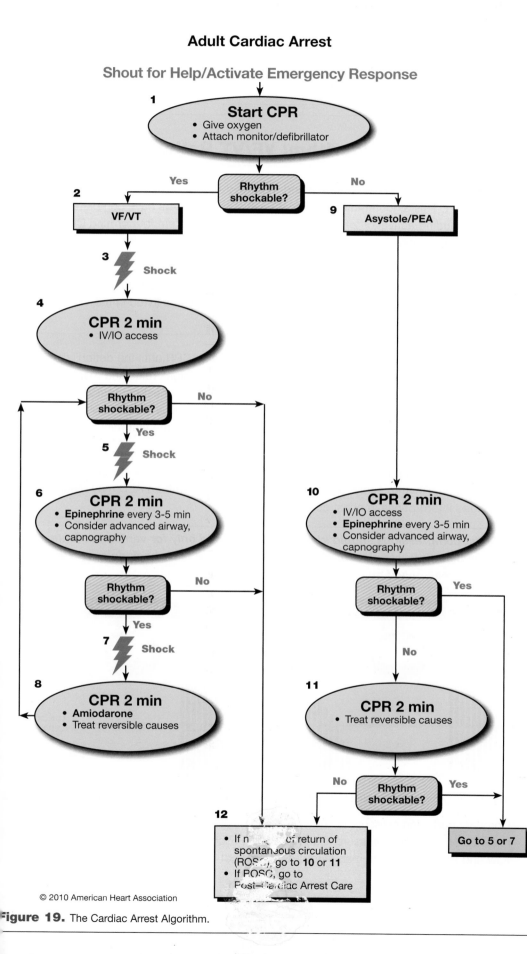

Adult Cardiac Arrest

Shout for Help/Activate Emergency Response

1 Start CPR
• Give oxygen
• Attach monitor/defibrillator

Rhythm shockable?

Yes → **2 VF/VT**
No → **9 Asystole/PEA**

3 Shock

4 CPR 2 min
• IV/IO access

Rhythm shockable?
No →
Yes ↓

5 Shock

6 CPR 2 min
• **Epinephrine** every 3-5 min
• Consider advanced airway, capnography

Rhythm shockable?
No →
Yes ↓

7 Shock

8 CPR 2 min
• **Amiodarone**
• Treat reversible causes

10 CPR 2 min
• IV/IO access
• **Epinephrine** every 3-5 min
• Consider advanced airway, capnography

Rhythm shockable?
Yes →
No ↓

11 CPR 2 min
• Treat reversible causes

Rhythm shockable?
No →
Yes →

12
• If no signs of return of spontaneous circulation (ROSC), go to **10** or **11**
• If ROSC, go to Post–Cardiac Arrest Care

Go to 5 or 7

© 2010 American Heart Association

Figure 19. The Cardiac Arrest Algorithm.

CPR Quality
• Push hard (≥5 cm [2 inches]) and fast (≥100/min) and allow complete chest recoil
• Minimize interruptions in compressions
• Avoid excessive ventilation
• Rotate compressor every 2 minutes
• If no advanced airway, 30:2 compression-ventilation ratio
• Quantitative waveform capnography
  – If P_{ETCO_2} <10 mm Hg, attempt to improve CPR quality
• Intra-arterial pressure
  – If relaxation phase (diastolic) pressure <20 mm Hg, attempt to improve CPR quality

Return of Spontaneous Circulation (ROSC)
• Pulse and blood pressure
• Abrupt sustained increase in P_{ETCO_2} (typically ≥40 mm Hg)
• Spontaneous arterial pressure waves with intra-arterial monitoring

Shock Energy
• **Biphasic:** Manufacturer recommendation (e.g., initial dose of 120-200 J); if unknown, use maximum available. Second and subsequent doses should be equivalent, and higher doses may be considered.
• **Monophasic:** 360 J

Drug Therapy
• **Epinephrine IV/IO Dose:** 1 mg every 3-5 minutes
• **Vasopressin IV/IO Dose:** 40 units can replace first or second dose of epinephrine
• **Amiodarone IV/IO Dose:** First dose: 300 mg bolus. Second dose: 150 mg.

Advanced Airway
• Supraglottic advanced airway or endotracheal intubation
• Waveform capnography to confirm and monitor ET tube placement
• 8-10 breaths per minute with continuous chest compressions

Reversible Causes
– **H**ypovolemia
– **H**ypoxia
– **H**ydrogen ion (acidosis)
– **H**ypo-/hyperkalemia
– **H**ypothermia
– **T**ension pneumothorax
– **T**amponade, cardiac
– **T**oxins
– **T**hrombosis, pulmonary
– **T**hrombosis, coronary

- The 2010 Cardiac Arrest Algorithms (Figures 19 and 21) are presented in the traditional box-and-line format and a new circular format (Figure 21). The 2 formats facilitate learning and memorization of the treatment recommendations. Overall these algorithms reflect an emphasis on the importance of high-quality, minimally interrupted CPR. This action is fundamental to the management of all cardiac arrest rhythms.

Application of the Cardiac Arrest Algorithm: VF/VT Pathway

Introduction (Boxes 1 Through 4)

This case discusses the assessment and treatment of a patient with refractory VF or pulseless VT. This algorithm assumes that healthcare providers have completed the BLS Survey, including activation of the emergency response system, performing CPR, attaching the manual defibrillator, and delivering the first shock (Boxes 1 through 4).

The ACLS resuscitation team now intervenes and conducts the ACLS Survey. In this case the team assesses the patient and takes actions as needed. The team leader coordinates the efforts of the resuscitation team as they perform the steps listed in the VF/VT pathway on the left side of the Cardiac Arrest Algorithm.

Minimal Interruption of Chest Compressions

A team member should continue to perform high-quality CPR until the defibrillator arrives and is attached to the patient. The team leader assigns roles and responsibilities and organizes interventions to minimize interruptions in chest compressions. This accomplishes the most critical interventions for VF or pulseless VT: CPR with minimal interruptions in chest compressions and defibrillation during the first minutes of arrest.

HSFC does not recommend continued use of an AED (or the automatic mode) when a manual defibrillator is available and the provider's skills are adequate for rhythm interpretation. Rhythm analysis and shock administration with an AED may result in prolonged interruptions in chest compressions.

> Chest compressions should ideally be interrupted only for ventilation (unless an advanced airway is placed), rhythm checks, and actual shock delivery. Perform a pulse check only if an organized rhythm is observed.

Figure 20. Relationship of quality CPR to coronary perfusion pressure (CPP) demonstrating the need to minimize interruptions in compressions.

Coronary perfusion pressure is aortic relaxation ("diastolic") pressure minus right atrial relaxation ("diastolic") pressure. During CPR, CPP correlates with both myocardial blood flow and ROSC. In one human study ROSC did not occur unless a CPP ≥15 mm Hg was achieved during CPR.

Foundational Facts **Resume CPR While Manual Defibrillator Is Charging**	• Shortening the interval between the last compression and the shock by even a few seconds can improve shock success (defibrillation and ROSC). Thus, it is reasonable for healthcare providers to practice efficient coordination between CPR and defibrillation to minimize the hands-off interval between stopping compressions and administering the shock. • For example, after verifying a shockable rhythm and initiating the charging sequence on the defibrillator, another rescuer should resume chest compressions and continue until the defibrillator is fully charged. The defibrillator operator should deliver the shock as soon as the compressor removes his or her hands from the patient's chest and all providers are "clear" of contact with the patient. • Use of a multimodal defibrillator in manual mode may reduce the duration of chest compression interruption required for rhythm analysis compared with automatic mode but could increase the frequency of inappropriate shock. Individuals who are not comfortable interpreting cardiac rhythms can continue to use an AED. • For an AED, follow the device's prompts.

Deliver 1 Shock (Box 3)

Box 3 directs you to deliver 1 shock. The appropriate energy dose is determined by the identity of the defibrillator—monophasic or biphasic. See the column on the right of the algorithm.

If you are using a *monophasic* defibrillator, give a single 360-J shock. Use the same energy dose for subsequent shocks.

Biphasic defibrillators use a variety of waveforms, each of which is effective for terminating VF over a specific dose range. When using biphasic defibrillators, providers should use the manufacturer's recommended energy dose (e.g., initial dose of 120 to 200 J). Many biphasic defibrillator manufacturers display the effective energy dose range on the face of the device. If you do not know the effective dose range, deliver the maximal energy dose for the first and all subsequent shocks.

If the initial shock terminates VF but the arrhythmia recurs later in the resuscitation attempt, deliver subsequent shocks at the previously successful energy level.

> *Immediately after the shock, resume CPR, beginning with chest compressions. Give 2 minutes (about 5 cycles) of CPR. A cycle consists of 30 compressions followed by 2 ventilations in the patient without an advanced airway.*

Resume CPR (Box 4)

• Immediately resume CPR, beginning with chest compressions.
• Do not perform a rhythm or pulse check at this point.
• Establish IV/IO access.

Foundational Facts
Clearing for Defibrillation

To ensure safety during defibrillation, always announce the shock warning. State the warning firmly and in a forceful voice before delivering each shock (this entire sequence should take <5 seconds):

- **"Clear. I am going to shock on three."**
  - Check to make sure you are clear of contact with the patient, the stretcher, or other equipment.
  - Make a visual check to ensure that no one is touching the patient or stretcher.
  - Be sure oxygen is not flowing across the patient's chest.
- **"One, two, three. Shocking."** When pressing the SHOCK button, the defibrillator operator should face the patient, not the machine. This helps to ensure coordination with the chest compressor and to verify that no one resumed contact with the patient.

You need not use these exact words, but you must warn others that you are about to deliver shocks and that everyone must stand clear of the patient.

Rhythm Check (Boxes 5 and 12)

Box 5 directs you to conduct a rhythm check after 2 minutes (about 5 cycles) of CPR. Be careful to minimize interruptions in chest compressions.

> *The pause in chest compressions to check the rhythm should not exceed 10 seconds.*

- If a nonshockable rhythm is present and the rhythm is organized (regular and narrow complexes), a team member should try to palpate a pulse. If there is any doubt about the presence of a pulse, immediately resume CPR.
- **Remember:** *Perform a pulse check—preferably during rhythm analysis—only if an organized rhythm is present.*
- If the rhythm is organized and there is a palpable pulse, proceed to post–cardiac arrest care.
- If the rhythm check reveals a nonshockable rhythm and there is no pulse, proceed along the asystole/PEA pathway on the right side of the Cardiac Arrest Algorithm (Boxes 9 through 11).
- If the rhythm check reveals a shockable rhythm, give 1 shock and resume CPR immediately for 2 minutes after the shock (Box 6).

Foundational Facts
Paddles vs Pads

- Using conductive materials during the defibrillation attempt reduces transthoracic impedance, or the resistance that chest structures have on electrical current.
- Conductive materials include paddles with electrode paste, gel pads, or self-adhesive pads.
- No existing data suggest that one is better than the others. Self-adhesive pads, however, reduce the risk of arcing, allow monitoring of the patient's underlying rhythm, and permit the rapid delivery of a shock if necessary.

For these reasons, HSFC recommends routine use of self-adhesive pads instead of paddles.

Shock and Vasopressors (Box 6)

For persistent VF/pulseless VT, give 1 shock and resume CPR immediately for 2 minutes (about 5 cycles) after the shock.

> *Immediately after the shock, resume CPR, beginning with chest compressions. Give 2 minutes (about 5 cycles) of CPR.*

When IV/IO access is available, give a vasopressor during CPR (either before or after the shock) as follows:

- **Epinephrine** 1 mg IV/IO—repeat every 3 to 5 minutes

or

- **Vasopressin** 40 units IV/IO—may substitute for the first or second dose of epinephrine

Note: If additional team members are available, they should anticipate the need for drugs and prepare them in advance.

Epinephrine hydrochloride is used during resuscitation primarily for its α-adrenergic effects, i.e., vasoconstriction. Vasoconstriction increases cerebral and coronary blood flow during CPR by increasing mean arterial pressure and aortic diastolic pressure. In previous studies, escalating and high-dose epinephrine administration did not improve survival to discharge or neurologic outcome after resuscitation from cardiac arrest.

Vasopressin is a nonadrenergic peripheral vasoconstrictor. A meta-analysis of 5 randomized trials found no difference between vasopressin and epinephrine for ROSC, 24-hour survival, or survival to hospital discharge.

Rhythm Check (Box 7)

Box 7 directs you to conduct a rhythm check after 2 minutes (about 5 cycles) of CPR. Be careful to minimize interruptions in chest compressions.

> *Interruption in CPR to conduct a rhythm analysis should not exceed 10 seconds.*

- If a nonshockable rhythm is present and the rhythm is organized (regular and narrow complexes), a team member should try to palpate a pulse. If there is any doubt about the presence of a pulse, immediately resume CPR.
- If the rhythm check is organized and there is a palpable pulse, proceed to post–cardiac arrest care.
- If the rhythm check reveals a nonshockable rhythm and there is no pulse, proceed along the asystole/PEA pathway on the right side of the Cardiac Arrest Algorithm (Boxes 9 through 11).
- If the rhythm check reveals a shockable rhythm, resume chest compressions if indicated while the defibrillator is charging (Box 8). The team leader is responsible for team safety while compressions are being performed and the defibrillator is charging.

Shock and Antiarrhythmics (Box 8)

Give 1 shock and resume CPR beginning with chest compressions for 2 minutes (about 5 cycles) immediately after the shock.

Healthcare providers may consider giving antiarrhythmic drugs, either before or after the shock; however, there is no evidence that any antiarrhythmic drug given during cardiac arrest increases survival to hospital discharge. If administered, amiodarone is the first-line antiarrhythmic agent given in cardiac arrest because it has been clinically demonstrated that it improves the rate of ROSC and hospital admission in adults with refractory VF/pulseless VT.

- **Amiodarone** 300 mg IV/IO bolus, then consider an additional 150 mg IV/IO once

If amiodarone is not available, providers may administer lidocaine.

- **Lidocaine** 1 to 1.5 mg/kg IV/IO first dose, then 0.5 to 0.75 mg/kg IV/IO at 5- to 10-minute intervals, to a maximum dose of 3 mg/kg

Providers should consider magnesium sulfate only for torsades de pointes associated with a long QT interval.

- **Magnesium sulfate** for torsades de pointes, loading dose 1 to 2 g IV/IO diluted in 10 mL of D_5W given as IV/IO bolus, typically over 5 to 20 minutes

Routine administration of magnesium sulfate in cardiac arrest is not recommended unless torsades de pointes is present.

Search for and treat any treatable underlying cause of cardiac arrest. See column on the right of the algorithm.

Cardiac Arrest Treatment Sequences

The Cardiac Arrest Circular Algorithm (Figure 21) summarizes the recommended sequence of CPR, rhythm checks, shocks, and delivery of drugs based on expert consensus. The optimal number of cycles of CPR and shocks required before starting pharmacologic therapy remains unknown. Note that rhythm checks and shocks are organized around 5 cycles of compressions and ventilations, or 2 minutes if a provider is timing the arrest.

Adult Cardiac Arrest

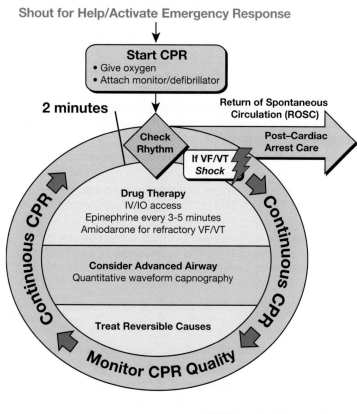

CPR Quality
- Push hard (≥5 cm [2 inches]) and fast (≥100/min) and allow complete chest recoil
- Minimize interruptions in compressions
- Avoid excessive ventilation
- Rotate compressor every 2 minutes
- If no advanced airway, 30:2 compression-ventilation ratio
- Quantitative waveform capnography
  - If PETCO$_2$ <10 mm Hg, attempt to improve CPR quality
- Intra-arterial pressure
  - If relaxation phase (diastolic) pressure <20 mm Hg, attempt to improve CPR quality

Return of Spontaneous Circulation (ROSC)
- Pulse and blood pressure
- Abrupt sustained increase in PETCO$_2$ (typically ≥40 mm Hg)
- Spontaneous arterial pressure waves with intra-arterial monitoring

Shock Energy
- **Biphasic:** Manufacturer recommendation (e.g., initial dose of 120-200 J); if unknown, use maximum available. Second and subsequent doses should be equivalent, and higher doses may be considered.
- **Monophasic:** 360 J

Drug Therapy
- **Epinephrine IV/IO Dose:** 1 mg every 3-5 minutes
- **Vasopressin IV/IO Dose:** 40 units can replace first or second dose of epinephrine
- **Amiodarone IV/IO Dose:** First dose: 300 mg bolus. Second dose: 150 mg.

Advanced Airway
- Supraglottic advanced airway or endotracheal intubation
- Waveform capnography to confirm and monitor ET tube placement
- 8-10 breaths per minute with continuous chest compressions

Reversible Causes
- Hypovolemia
- Hypoxia
- Hydrogen ion (acidosis)
- Hypo-/hyperkalemia
- Hypothermia
- Tension pneumothorax
- Tamponade, cardiac
- Toxins
- Thrombosis, pulmonary
- Thrombosis, coronary

© 2010 American Heart Association

Figure 21. The Cardiac Arrest Circular Algorithm. Do not delay shock. Continue CPR while preparing and administering drugs and charging the defibrillator. Interrupt chest compressions only for the minimum amount of time required for ventilation (until advanced airway placed), rhythm check, and actual shock delivery.

<table>
<tr>
<td>

FYI 2010 Guidelines

Cardiac Arrest Circular Algorithm

</td>
<td>

- The *2010 Guidelines for CPR and ECC* introduced a new circular format for the Cardiac Arrest Algorithm (Figure 21) to facilitate learning and memorization of the treatment recommendations. This new algorithm emphasizes the importance of high-quality, minimally interrupted CPR, which is fundamental to the management of all cardiac arrest rhythms.

</td>
</tr>
</table>

Physiologic Monitoring During CPR

The *2010 Guidelines for CPR and ECC* recommend using quantitative waveform capnography in intubated patients to monitor CPR quality (Figure 22A), optimize chest compressions, and detect ROSC during chest compressions (Figure 23) or when rhythm check reveals an organized rhythm. Although placement of invasive monitors during CPR is not generally warranted, physiologic parameters such as intra-arterial relaxation pressures (Figure 22A) and central venous oxygen saturation ($ScvO_2$), when available, may also be helpful for optimizing CPR and detecting ROSC.

Animal and human studies indicate that $PETCO_2$, CPP, and $ScvO_2$ monitoring provides valuable information on both the patient's condition and the response to therapy. Most important, $PETCO_2$, CPP, and $ScvO_2$ correlate with cardiac output and myocardial blood flow during CPR. When chest compressions fail to achieve identified threshold values, ROSC is rarely achieved. Furthermore, an abrupt increase in any of these parameters is a sensitive indicator of ROSC that can be monitored without interrupting chest compressions.

Although no clinical study has examined whether titrating resuscitative efforts to physiologic parameters improves outcome, it is reasonable to use these parameters, if available, to optimize compressions and guide vasopressor therapy during cardiac arrest.

End-Tidal CO_2

The main determinant of $PETCO_2$ during CPR is blood delivery to the lungs. Persistently low $PETCO_2$ values <10 mm Hg during CPR in intubated patients (Figure 22B) suggest that ROSC is unlikely. If $PETCO_2$ abruptly increases to a normal value of 35 to 40 mm Hg, it is reasonable to consider this an indicator of ROSC.

- If the $PETCO_2$ is <10 mm Hg during CPR, it is reasonable to try to improve chest compressions and vasopressor therapy.

Coronary Perfusion Pressure or Arterial Relaxation Pressure (if available)

Increased CPP correlates with both myocardial blood flow and ROSC. A reasonable surrogate for CPP during CPR is arterial relaxation ("diastolic") pressure, which can be measured by using an intra-arterial catheter.

- If the arterial relaxation pressure is <20 mm Hg (Figure 22B), it is reasonable to try to improve chest compressions and vasopressor therapy.

Central Venous Oxygen Saturation

If oxygen consumption, arterial oxygen saturation, and hemoglobin are constant, changes in $ScvO_2$ reflect changes in oxygen delivery due to changes in cardiac output. $ScvO_2$ can be measured continuously by using oximetric tipped central venous catheters placed in the superior vena cava or pulmonary artery. Normal range is 60% to 80%.

- If the $ScvO_2$ is <30%, it is reasonable to try to improve chest compressions and vasopressor therapy.

Figure 22. Physiologic monitoring during CPR. **A.** High-quality compressions are shown through waveform capnography and intra-arterial relaxation pressure. PETCO₂ values <10 mm Hg in intubated patients or intra-arterial relaxation pressures <20 mm Hg indicate that cardiac output is inadequate to achieve ROSC. In either of those cases it is reasonable to consider trying to improve quality of CPR by optimizing chest compression parameters or giving a vasopressor or both. **B.** Ineffective CPR compressions shown through waveform capnography and intra-arterial relaxation pressure.

Figure 23. Waveform capnography during CPR with ROSC. This capnography tracing displays P_{ETCO_2} in millimeters of mercury on the vertical axis over time. This patient is intubated and receiving CPR. Note that the ventilation rate is approximately 8 to 10 breaths per minute. Chest compressions are given continuously at a rate slightly faster than 100/min but are not visible with this tracing. The initial P_{ETCO_2} is <12.5 mm Hg during the first minute, indicating very low blood flow. P_{ETCO_2} increases to between 12.5 and 25 mm Hg during the second and third minutes, consistent with the increase in blood flow with ongoing resuscitation. ROSC occurs during the fourth minute. ROSC is recognized by the abrupt increase in P_{ETCO_2} (visible just after the fourth vertical line) to >50 mm Hg, which is consistent with a substantial improvement in blood flow.

Treatment of VF/VT in Hypothermia

For a cardiac arrest patient in VF/VT who has severe hypothermia and a body temperature of <30°C (<86°F), a single defibrillation attempt is appropriate. If the patient fails to respond to the initial shock, it is reasonable to perform additional defibrillation attempts according to the usual BLS guidelines while engaging in active rewarming. The hypothermic patient may have a reduced rate of drug metabolism, raising concern that drug levels may accumulate to toxic levels with standard dosing regimens. Although the evidence does not support the use of antiarrhythmic drug therapy in hypothermic patients in cardiac arrest, it is reasonable to consider administration of a vasopressor according to the standard ACLS algorithm concurrent with rewarming strategies.

ACLS treatment of the patient with severe hypothermia in cardiac arrest in the hospital should be aimed at rapid core rewarming.

For patients in cardiac arrest with moderate hypothermia (30°C to 34°C [86°F to 93.2°F]), start CPR, attempt defibrillation, give medications spaced at longer intervals, and, if in hospital, provide active core rewarming.

Routes of Access for Drugs

Priorities

Priorities during cardiac arrest are high-quality CPR and early defibrillation. Insertion of an advanced airway and drug administration are of secondary importance. No drug given during cardiac arrest has been shown to improve survival to hospital discharge or improve neurologic function after cardiac arrest.

Historically in ACLS, providers have administered drugs via either the IV or endotracheal route. Endotracheal absorption of drugs is poor and optimal drug dosing is not known. For this reason, the IO route is preferred when IV access is not available. Priorities for vascular access are:

- IV route
- IO route
- Endotracheal route

Intravenous Route

A peripheral IV is preferred for drug and fluid administration unless central line access is already available.

Central line access is not necessary during most resuscitation attempts. Central line access may cause interruptions in CPR and complications during insertion, including vascular laceration, hematomas, and bleeding. Insertion of a central line noncompressible vessel is a relative (not absolute) contraindication to fibrinolytic therapy in patients with ACS.

Establishing a peripheral line does not require interruption of CPR. Drugs, however, typically require 1 to 2 minutes to reach the central circulation when given by the peripheral IV route. Keep in mind that drugs administered during the CPR sequence will likely not take effect until completion of several cycles of CPR.

If a drug is given by the peripheral venous route, administer it as follows:

- Give the drug by bolus injection unless otherwise specified.
- Follow with a 20-mL bolus of IV fluid.
- Elevate the extremity for about 10 to 20 seconds to facilitate delivery of the drug to the central circulation.

Intraosseous Route

Drugs and fluids during resuscitation can be delivered safely and effectively via the IO route if IV access is not available. Important points about IO access are:

- IO access can be established in all age groups.
- IO access often can be achieved in 30 to 60 seconds.
- The IO route of administration is preferred over the endotracheal route.
- Any ACLS drug or fluid that is administered IV can be given IO.

IO cannulation provides access to a noncollapsible marrow venous plexus, which serves as a rapid, safe, and reliable route for administration of drugs, crystalloids, colloids, and blood during resuscitation. The technique uses a rigid needle, preferably a specially designed IO or bone marrow needle from an IO access kit.

Endotracheal Route

IV and IO administration routes are preferred over the endotracheal administration route. When considering administration of drugs via the endotracheal route during CPR, keep these concepts in mind:

- The optimal dose of most drugs given by the endotracheal route is unknown.
- The typical dose of drugs administered via the endotracheal route is 2 to 2½ times the IV route.

Studies demonstrate that epinephrine, vasopressin, and lidocaine are absorbed into the circulatory system after administration via the endotracheal route. When giving drugs via the endotracheal route, dilute the dose in 5 to 10 mL of sterile water or normal saline. Inject the drug directly into the trachea.

Vasopressors

Introduction

There is no evidence to date that routine use of any vasopressor at any stage during management of cardiac arrest increases rates of survival to hospital discharge. But there is evidence that the use of vasopressors favors initial resuscitation with ROSC.

Vasopressors Used During Cardiac Arrest

Vasopressors optimize cardiac output and blood pressure. The vasopressors used during cardiac arrest are:

- Epinephrine: 1 mg IV/IO (repeat every 3 to 5 minutes)
- Vasopressin: 1 dose of 40 units IV/IO may replace either the first or second dose of epinephrine

If IV/IO access cannot be established or is delayed, give epinephrine 2 to 2.5 mg diluted in 5 to 10 mL of sterile water or normal saline and injected directly into the ET tube. Remember, the endotracheal route of drug administration results in variable and unpredictable drug absorption and blood levels.

Epinephrine

Although healthcare providers have used epinephrine for years in resuscitation, there are few data to show that it improves outcome in humans. Epinephrine administration does appear to improve ROSC. No studies demonstrate improved rates of survival to hospital discharge or neurologic outcome when comparing standard epinephrine doses with initial high-dose or escalating dose epinephrine. Therefore, HSFC cannot recommend the routine use of high-dose or escalating doses of epinephrine.

Epinephrine is thought to stimulate adrenergic receptors, producing vasoconstriction, increasing blood pressure and heart rate, and improving perfusion pressure to the brain and heart.

Repeat epinephrine 1 mg IV/IO every 3 to 5 minutes during cardiac arrest.

> *Remember, follow each dose given by peripheral injection with a 20-mL flush of IV fluid and elevate the extremity above the level of the heart for 10 to 20 seconds.*

Vasopressin

Vasopressin is a nonadrenergic peripheral vasoconstrictor that increases arterial blood pressure. Because the efficacy of vasopressin is no different from that of epinephrine in cardiac arrest, a single dose of vasopressin (40 units IV/IO) may replace either the first or second dose of epinephrine.

Foundational Facts
Vasopressors

Because the effects of vasopressin have not been shown to differ from those of epinephrine in cardiac arrest, either vasopressin or epinephrine can be used as the initial vasopressor during cardiac arrest.

- A vasopressor is given every 3 to 5 minutes during cardiac arrest.
- One dose of vasopressin 40 units IV/IO may replace either the first or second dose of epinephrine in the treatment of cardiac arrest.
- Epinephrine is administered 3 to 5 minutes after the dose of vasopressin if there is a continuing need for a vasopressor.

Antiarrhythmic Agents

Introduction

There is no evidence that any antiarrhythmic drug given routinely during human cardiac arrest increases survival to hospital discharge. Amiodarone, however, has been shown to increase short-term survival to hospital admission when compared with placebo or lidocaine.

Amiodarone

- Consider amiodarone for treatment of VF or pulseless VT unresponsive to shock delivery, CPR, and a vasopressor.
- Amiodarone is a complex drug that affects sodium, potassium, and calcium channels. It also has α-adrenergic and β-adrenergic blocking properties.
- During cardiac arrest, consider amiodarone 300 mg IV/IO push for the first dose. If VF/pulseless VT persists, consider giving a second dose of 150 mg IV/IO in 3 to 5 minutes.

Lidocaine

- Lidocaine is an alternative antiarrhythmic of long-standing and widespread familiarity. However, it has no proven short-term or long-term efficacy in cardiac arrest. Providers may consider giving lidocaine when amiodarone is not available.
- The initial lidocaine dose is 1 to 1.5 mg/kg IV/IO. Repeat if indicated at 0.5 to 0.75 mg/kg IV/IO over 5- to 10-minute intervals to a maximum of 3 mg/kg.
- If no IV/IO access is available, the dose for endotracheal administration is 2 to 4 mg/kg.

Magnesium Sulfate

- IV magnesium may terminate or prevent recurrent torsades de pointes in patients who have a prolonged QT interval during normal sinus rhythm. When VF/pulseless VT cardiac arrest is associated with torsades de pointes, give magnesium sulfate at a loading dose of 1 to 2 g IV/IO diluted in 10 mL D_5W given over 5 to 20 minutes. If a prearrest 12-lead ECG is available for review, check the QT interval for prolongation.
- Remember that pulseless VT is treated with an immediate high-energy shock, whereas magnesium is an adjunctive agent used to *prevent* recurrent or treat persistent VT associated with torsades de pointes.
- Magnesium sulfate is also indicated for patients with known or suspected low serum magnesium, such as patients with alcoholism or other conditions associated with malnutrition or hypomagnesemic states. For patients in refractory VF/pulseless VT, check the patient's history, if available, for one of these conditions that suggests the presence of a reversible electrolyte abnormality.

Immediate Post–Cardiac Arrest Care

Introduction

There is increasing recognition that systematic post–cardiac arrest care after ROSC can improve the likelihood of patient survival with good quality of life. This case focuses on the management of and optimization of cardiopulmonary function and perfusion of vital organs after ROSC.

To ensure the success of post–cardiac arrest care, healthcare providers must:

- Optimize the patient's hemodynamic and ventilation status
- Initiate therapeutic hypothermia
- Provide immediate coronary reperfusion with PCI
- Institute glycemic control
- Provide neurologic care and prognostication and other structured interventions

In this case you will have an opportunity to use the 12-lead ECG while using the assessment and action skills typically performed after ROSC.

Managing Post–Cardiac Arrest Care: The Post–Cardiac Arrest Care Algorithm

The Immediate Post–Cardiac Arrest Care Algorithm (Figure 24) outlines all the steps for immediate assessment and management of post–cardiac arrest patients with ROSC. During this case team members will continue to maintain good ventilation and oxygenation with a bag-mask device or advanced airway. Throughout the case discussion of the Post–Cardiac Arrest Care Algorithm, we will refer to Boxes 1 through 8. These are the numbers assigned to the boxes on the algorithm.

Adult Immediate Post–Cardiac Arrest Care

1
Return of Spontaneous Circulation (ROSC)

2
Optimize ventilation and oxygenation
- Maintain oxygen saturation ≥94%
- Consider advanced airway and waveform capnography
- Do not hyperventilate

3
Treat hypotension (SBP <90 mm Hg)
- IV/IO bolus
- Vasopressor infusion
- Consider treatable causes
- 12-Lead ECG

4
Follow commands?

5
Consider induced hypothermia — No

6
STEMI OR high suspicion of AMI — Yes

7
Coronary reperfusion — Yes

8
Advanced critical care

Doses/Details

Ventilation/Oxygenation
Avoid excessive ventilation. Start at 10-12 breaths/min and titrate to target PETCO$_2$ of 35-40 mm Hg. When feasible, titrate FIO$_2$ to minimum necessary to achieve SpO$_2$ ≥94%.

IV Bolus
1-2 L normal saline or lactated Ringer's. If inducing hypothermia, may use 4°C fluid.

Epinephrine IV Infusion:
0.1-0.5 mcg/kg per minute (in 70-kg adult: 7-35 mcg per minute)

Dopamine IV Infusion:
5-10 mcg/kg per minute

Norepinephrine IV Infusion:
0.1-0.5 mcg/kg per minute (in 70-kg adult: 7-35 mcg per minute)

Reversible Causes
- Hypovolemia
- Hypoxia
- Hydrogen ion (acidosis)
- Hypo-/hyperkalemia
- Hypothermia
- Tension pneumothorax
- Tamponade, cardiac
- Toxins
- Thrombosis, pulmonary
- Thrombosis, coronary

© 2010 American Heart Association

Figure 24. The Immediate Post–Cardiac Arrest Care Algorithm.

Application of the Immediate Post–Cardiac Arrest Care Algorithm

Introduction (Box 1)   This case discusses the assessment and treatment of a patient who had cardiac arrest and was resuscitated with the use of the BLS Survey and ACLS Survey. During rhythm check in the ACLS Survey, the patient's rhythm was organized and a pulse was detected (Box 12, Cardiac Arrest Algorithm [Figure 19]). The team leader will coordinate the efforts of the post–cardiac arrest care team as they perform the steps of the Post–Cardiac Arrest Care Algorithm.

Optimize Ventilation and Oxygenation (Box 2)

Box 2 directs you to ensure an adequate airway and support breathing immediately after ROSC. An unconscious/unresponsive patient will require an advanced airway for mechanical support of breathing.

- Use continuous waveform capnography to confirm and monitor correct placement of the ET tube (Figures 25 and 26).
- Use the lowest inspired oxygen concentration that will maintain arterial oxyhemoglobin saturation ≥94%. When titration of inspired oxygen is not feasible (e.g., in an out-of-hospital setting), it is reasonable to empirically use 100% oxygen until the patient arrives at the ED.
- Avoid excessive ventilation of the patient (do not ventilate too fast or too much). Providers may begin ventilations at 10 to 12 breaths per minute and titrate to achieve a P_{ETCO_2} of 35 to 40 mm Hg or a $Paco_2$ of 40 to 45 mm Hg.

If appropriate equipment is available, adjust the FIO_2 after achieving ROSC to the minimum concentration needed to achieve arterial oxyhemoglobin saturation ≥94%. The goal is to avoid hyperoxia while ensuring adequate oxygen delivery.

Because an oxygen saturation of 100% may correspond to a Pao_2 between approximately 80 and 500 mm Hg, in general it is appropriate to wean FIO_2 for a saturation of 100%, provided the patient can maintain oxyhemoglobin saturation ≥94%.

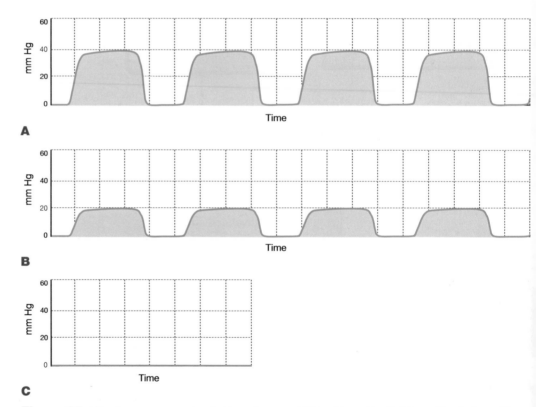

Figure 25. Waveform capnography. **A.** Normal range of 35 to 45 mm Hg. **B.** 20 mm Hg. **C.** 0 mm Hg.

Figure 26. Waveform capnography with an ET tube, showing normal (adequate) ventilation pattern: PETCO₂ 35 to 40 mm Hg

Critical Concepts **Waveform Capnography**	• In addition to monitoring ET tube position, quantitative waveform capnography allows healthcare personnel to monitor CPR quality, optimize chest compressions, and detect ROSC during chest compressions or when a rhythm check reveals an organized rhythm.

Caution **Things to Avoid During Ventilation**	• When securing an advanced airway, avoid using ties that pass circumferentially around the patient's neck, thereby obstructing venous return from the brain. • Excessive ventilation may potentially lead to adverse hemodynamic effects when intrathoracic pressures are increased and because of potential decreases in cerebral blood flow when PaCO₂ decreases.

- End-tidal CO_2 is the concentration of carbon dioxide in exhaled air at the end of expiration. It is typically expressed as a partial pressure in millimeters of mercury (P_{ETCO_2}). Because CO_2 is a trace gas in atmospheric air, CO_2 detected by capnography in exhaled air is produced in the body and delivered to the lungs by circulating blood.
- Cardiac output is the major determinant of CO_2 delivery to the lungs. If ventilation is relatively constant, P_{ETCO_2} correlates well with cardiac output during CPR.
- Providers should observe a persistent capnographic waveform with ventilation to confirm and monitor ET tube placement in the field, in the transport vehicle, on arrival at the hospital, and after any patient transfer to reduce the risk of unrecognized tube misplacement or displacement.
- Although capnography to confirm and monitor correct placement of supraglottic airways (e.g., laryngeal mask airway, laryngeal tube, or esophageal-tracheal tube) has not been studied, effective ventilation through a supraglottic airway device should result in a capnography waveform during CPR and after ROSC.

- Continuous waveform capnography is recommended, in addition to clinical assessment, as the most reliable method of confirming and monitoring correct placement of an ET tube.

Treat Hypotension (SBP <90 mm Hg) (Box 3)

Box 3 directs you to treat hypotension when SBP is <90 mm Hg. Providers should obtain IV access if not already established. Verify the patency of any IV lines. IV lines should replace IO access if IO is used during resuscitation. ECG monitoring should continue after ROSC, during transport, and throughout ICU care until deemed clinically not necessary. At this stage, consider treating any reversible causes that might have precipitated the cardiac arrest but persist after ROSC.

When IV is established, treat hypotension as follows:

- **IV bolus** 1-2 L normal saline or lactated Ringer's. If therapeutic hypothermia is indicated or will be performed, you may use 4°C fluids.
- **Epinephrine** 0.1-0.5 mcg/kg per minute (in 70-kg adult: 7-35 mcg per minute) IV infusion titrated to achieve a minimum SBP of >90 mm Hg or a mean arterial pressure of >65 mm Hg
- **Dopamine** 5-10 mcg/kg per minute IV infusion titrated to achieve a minimum SBP of >90 mm Hg or a mean arterial pressure of >65 mm Hg
- **Norepinephrine** 0.1-0.5 mcg/kg per minute (in 70-kg adult: 7-35 mcg per minute) IV infusion titrated to achieve a minimum SBP of >90 mm Hg or a mean arterial pressure of >65 mm Hg

Epinephrine can be used in patients who are not in cardiac arrest but who require inotropic or vasopressor support.

Dopamine hydrochloride is a catecholamine-like agent and a chemical precursor of norepinephrine that stimulates the heart through both α- and β-adrenergic receptors.

Norepinephrine (levarterenol) is a naturally occurring potent vasoconstrictor and inotropic agent. It may be effective for management of patients with severe hypotension (e.g., SBP <70 mm Hg) and a low total peripheral resistance who fail to respond to less potent adrenergic drugs such as dopamine, phenylephrine, or methoxamine.

Following Commands (Box 4)

Box 4 directs you to examine the patient's ability to follow verbal commands.

If the patient fails to follow commands, the healthcare team should consider implementing therapeutic hypothermia (Box 5). If the patient is able to follow verbal commands, move to Box 6.

Therapeutic Hypothermia (Box 5)

To protect the brain and other organs, the resuscitation team should induce therapeutic hypothermia in adult patients who remain comatose (lack of meaningful response to verbal commands) with ROSC after out-of-hospital VF cardiac arrest. When ROSC occurs in the out-of-hospital setting, EMS personnel may initiate the cooling process and should transport the patient to a facility that reliably provides this therapy.

Healthcare providers should cool patients to a target temperature of 32°C to 34°C for a period of 12 to 24 hours. Although the optimal method of achieving the target temperature is unknown, any combination of rapid infusion of ice-cold, isotonic, non–glucose-containing fluid (30 mL/kg), endovascular catheters, surface cooling devices, or simple surface interventions (e.g., ice bags) appears safe and effective.

Healthcare providers should also consider induced hypothermia for comatose adult patients with ROSC after in-hospital cardiac arrest of any initial rhythm or after out-of-hospital cardiac arrest with an initial rhythm of PEA or asystole.

Caution
Avoid Active Rewarming After ROSC

- In comatose patients who spontaneously develop a mild degree of hypothermia (>32°C) after resuscitation from cardiac arrest, avoid active rewarming during the first 12 to 24 hours after ROSC.

Foundational Facts
Induced Hypothermia

- Therapeutic hypothermia is the only intervention demonstrated to improve neurologic recovery after cardiac arrest.
- The optimal duration of induced hypothermia is at least 12 hours and may be >24 hours. The effect of a longer duration of cooling on outcome has not been studied in adults, but hypothermia for up to 72 hours was used safely in newborns.
- Healthcare providers should monitor the patient's core temperature during induced hypothermia by using an esophageal thermometer, a bladder catheter in nonanuric patients, or a pulmonary artery catheter if one is placed for other indications. Axillary and oral temperatures are inadequate for measurement of core temperature changes.
- Induced hypothermia should not affect the decision to perform PCI, because concurrent PCI and hypothermia are reported to be feasible and safe.

STEMI Is Present or High Suspicion of AMI (Box 6)

Both in- and out-of-hospital medical personnel should obtain a 12-lead ECG as soon as possible after ROSC in order to identify those patients with STEMI or a high suspicion of AMI. Once identified, hospital personnel should attempt coronary reperfusion (Box 7). EMS personnel should transport these patients to a facility that reliably provides this therapy (Box 7).

Coronary Reperfusion (Box 7)

Aggressive treatment of STEMI or AMI should begin if detected after ROSC, regardless of coma or induced hypothermia, including coronary reperfusion with PCI. In the case of out-of-hospital STEMI, provide advance notification to receiving facilities for patients diagnosed with STEMI to reduce reperfusion delay.

Advanced Critical Care (Box 8)

Following coronary reperfusion interventions or in cases where the post–cardiac arrest patient has no ECG evidence or suspicion of MI, the healthcare team should transfer the patient to an intensive care unit.

Post–Cardiac Arrest Maintenance Therapy

There is no evidence to support continued prophylactic administration of antiarrhythmic medications once the patient achieves ROSC.

Pulseless Electrical Activity Case

Introduction

This case focuses on assessment and management of a *cardiac arrest patient with PEA*. During the BLS Survey, team members will demonstrate high-quality CPR with effective chest compressions and ventilation with a bag-mask. In the ACLS Survey the team leader will recognize PEA and implement the appropriate interventions outlined in the Cardiac Arrest Algorithm. Because correction of an underlying cause of PEA, if present and identified, is critical to patient outcome, the team leader will verbalize the differential diagnosis while leading the resuscitation team in the search for and treatment of reversible causes.

Learning Objectives

By the end of this case you should be able to:

1. Describe signs and symptoms of PEA

2. Demonstrate treatment priorities of individuals experiencing PEA as specified by the Cardiac Arrest Algorithm

3. State the correct dosage of epinephrine in PEA

4. Recall the correct method of administering epinephrine in PEA

5. State the correct dosage of vasopressin in PEA

6. Describe the target of PEA (treatment of the cause, not the rhythm)

7. Describe the most likely causes of PEA

8. Assign team functions, monitor CPR, monitor treatments, and monitor drug administration

Rhythms for PEA

You will need to recognize the following rhythms:

- Rate—too fast or too slow
- Width of QRS complexes—wide versus narrow

Drugs for PEA

This case involves these drugs:

- Epinephrine
- Vasopressin
- Other medications, depending on the cause of the PEA arrest

Description of PEA

Introduction

PEA encompasses a heterogeneous group of rhythms that are organized or semiorganized, but lack a palpable pulse. PEA includes:

- Idioventricular rhythms
- Ventricular escape rhythms
- Postdefibrillation idioventricular rhythms
- Sinus rhythm

Any organized rhythm without a pulse is defined as PEA. Even sinus rhythm without a detectable pulse is called PEA. Pulseless rhythms that are excluded by definition include VF, VT, and asystole.

Historical Perspective

Previously resuscitation teams used the term *electromechanical dissociation* (EMD) to describe patients who displayed electrical activity on the cardiac monitor but lacked apparent contractile function because of an undetectable pulse. That is, weak contractile function is present—detectable by invasive monitoring or echocardiography—but the cardiac function is too weak to produce a pulse or effective cardiac output. This is the most common initial condition present following successful defibrillation. PEA also includes other conditions where the heart is empty because of inadequate preload. In this case, the contractile function of the heart is adequate, but there is inadequate volume for the ventricle to eject. This may occur as a result of severe hypovolemia, or as a result of decreased venous return from pulmonary embolism or pneumothorax.

Managing PEA: The Cardiac Arrest Algorithm

Overview

As described earlier, the Cardiac Arrest Algorithm consists of 2 cardiac arrest pathways (Figures 19 and 27). The left side of the algorithm outlines treatment for a shockable rhythm (VF/VT). The right side of the algorithm (Boxes 9 through 11) outlines treatment for a nonshockable rhythm (asystole/PEA). Because of the similarity in causes and management, the Cardiac Arrest Algorithm combines the asystole and PEA pathways, although we will review these rhythms in separate cases. In both pathways, therapies are organized around periods (2 minutes or 5 cycles) of uninterrupted, high-quality CPR.

The ability to achieve a good resuscitation outcome with return of a perfusing rhythm and spontaneous respirations depends on the ability of the resuscitation team to provide effective CPR and to identify and correct a cause of PEA if present.

Everyone on the resuscitation team must carry out the steps outlined in the algorithm and at the same time focus on the identification and treatment of reversible causes of the arrest.

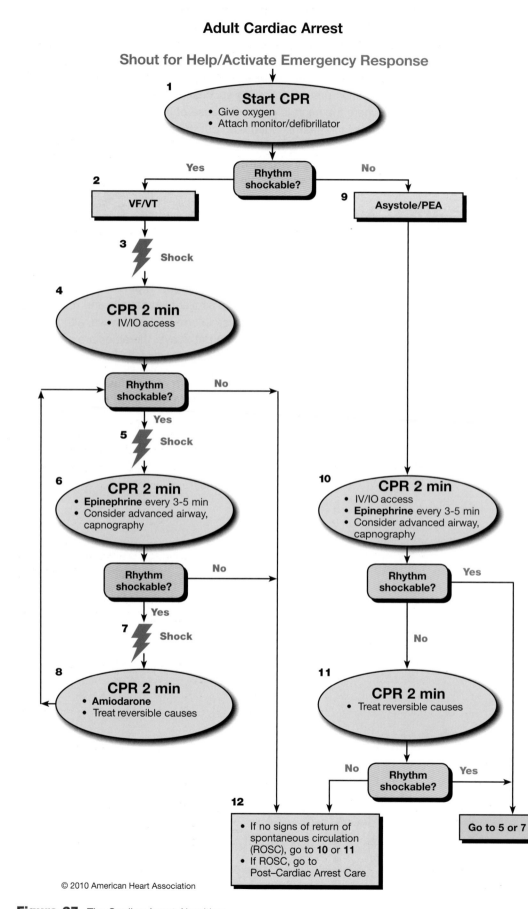

Adult Cardiac Arrest

Shout for Help/Activate Emergency Response

1 Start CPR
- Give oxygen
- Attach monitor/defibrillator

Rhythm shockable?

Yes → **2 VF/VT**

No → **9 Asystole/PEA**

3 Shock

4 CPR 2 min
- IV/IO access

Rhythm shockable?

No →

Yes ↓

5 Shock

6 CPR 2 min
- **Epinephrine** every 3-5 min
- Consider advanced airway, capnography

Rhythm shockable?

No →

Yes ↓

7 Shock

8 CPR 2 min
- **Amiodarone**
- Treat reversible causes

10 CPR 2 min
- IV/IO access
- **Epinephrine** every 3-5 min
- Consider advanced airway, capnography

Rhythm shockable?

Yes →

No ↓

11 CPR 2 min
- Treat reversible causes

Rhythm shockable?

No ←

Yes →

Go to 5 or 7

12
- If no signs of return of spontaneous circulation (ROSC), go to **10** or **11**
- If ROSC, go to Post–Cardiac Arrest Care

CPR Quality
- Push hard (≥5 cm [2 inches]) and fast (≥100/min) and allow complete chest recoil
- Minimize interruptions in compressions
- Avoid excessive ventilation
- Rotate compressor every 2 minutes
- If no advanced airway, 30:2 compression-ventilation ratio
- Quantitative waveform capnography
  - If P_{ETCO_2} <10 mm Hg, attempt to improve CPR quality
- Intra-arterial pressure
  - If relaxation phase (diastolic) pressure <20 mm Hg, attempt to improve CPR quality

Return of Spontaneous Circulation (ROSC)
- Pulse and blood pressure
- Abrupt sustained increase in P_{ETCO_2} (typically ≥40 mm Hg)
- Spontaneous arterial pressure waves with intra-arterial monitoring

Shock Energy
- **Biphasic:** Manufacturer recommendation (e.g., initial dose of 120-200 J); if unknown, use maximum available. Second and subsequent doses should be equivalent, and higher doses may be considered.
- **Monophasic:** 360 J

Drug Therapy
- **Epinephrine IV/IO Dose:** 1 mg every 3-5 minutes
- **Vasopressin IV/IO Dose:** 40 units can replace first or second dose of epinephrine
- **Amiodarone IV/IO Dose:** First dose: 300 mg bolus. Second dose: 150 mg.

Advanced Airway
- Supraglottic advanced airway or endotracheal intubation
- Waveform capnography to confirm and monitor ET tube placement
- 8-10 breaths per minute with continuous chest compressions

Reversible Causes
- **H**ypovolemia
- **H**ypoxia
- **H**ydrogen ion (acidosis)
- **H**ypo-/hyperkalemia
- **H**ypothermia
- **T**ension pneumothorax
- **T**amponade, cardiac
- **T**oxins
- **T**hrombosis, pulmonary
- **T**hrombosis, coronary

Figure 27. The Cardiac Arrest Algorithm.

The PEA Pathway of the Cardiac Arrest Algorithm

In this case the *patient is in cardiac arrest.* Team members initiate and perform high-quality CPR throughout the BLS Survey and the ACLS Survey. The team interrupts CPR for 10 seconds or less for rhythm and pulse checks. *This patient has an organized rhythm on the monitor but no pulse. The condition is PEA* (Box 9). Chest compressions resume immediately. The team leader now directs the team in the steps outlined in the PEA pathway of the Cardiac Arrest Algorithm (Figure 27), beginning with Box 10.

IV/IO access is a priority over advanced airway management unless bag-mask ventilation is ineffective or the arrest is caused by hypoxia. All resuscitation team members must simultaneously conduct a search for an underlying and treatable cause of the PEA in addition to performing their assigned roles.

Rhythm Check: Decision Point (Box 11)

Box 11 directs you to conduct a rhythm check and give 2 minutes (about 5 cycles) of CPR after administration of the drugs. Be careful to minimize interruptions in chest compressions.

> *The pause in CPR to conduct a rhythm check should not exceed 10 seconds.*

Administer Vasopressors (Box 10)

- Give a vasopressor as soon as IV/IO access becomes available.
  - Epinephrine 1 mg IV/IO—repeat every 3 to 5 minutes

or

  - Vasopressin 40 units IV/IO to replace first or second dose of epinephrine

> *Administer drugs during CPR. Do not stop CPR to administer drugs.*

No known vasopressor (epinephrine and vasopressin) increases survival from PEA. Because these medications can improve aortic diastolic blood pressure, coronary artery perfusion pressure, and the rate of ROSC, HSFC continues to recommend their use.

- Consider advanced airway and capnography.

FYI 2010 Guidelines

No Atropine During Cardiac Arrest

- There is no evidence that atropine has detrimental effects during bradycardic or asystolic cardiac arrest. On the other hand, available evidence suggests that routine use of atropine during PEA or asystole is unlikely to have a therapeutic benefit. For this reason, atropine has been removed from the Cardiac Arrest Algorithm.

Nonshockable Rhythm (Box 12)

- If *no electrical activity is present* (asystole), go back to Box 10.
- If organized electrical activity is present, try to palpate a pulse. Take at least 5 seconds but do not take more than 10 seconds to check for a pulse.
- If *no pulse is present*, or if there is any doubt about the presence of a pulse, immediately resume CPR for 2 minutes, starting with chest compressions. Go back to Box 10 and repeat the sequence.
- If a palpable pulse is present and the rhythm is organized, begin post–cardiac arrest care.

Decision Point: Shockable Rhythm (Box 12)

- If the rhythm check reveals a shockable rhythm, resume CPR with chest compressions while the defibrillator is charging if possible.
- Switch to the left side of the algorithm and perform steps according to the VF/VT sequence starting with Box 5 or 7.

3 easily Treated Causes
- hypoxia - hypovolemic   - Tension PTX

Asystole and PEA Treatment Sequences

Figure 28 summarizes the recommended sequence of CPR, rhythm checks, and delivery of drugs for PEA and asystole based on expert consensus.

Adult Cardiac Arrest

Shout for Help/Activate Emergency Response

Start CPR
- Give oxygen
- Attach monitor/defibrillator

2 minutes

Check Rhythm

Return of Spontaneous Circulation (ROSC)

If VF/VT Shock

Post–Cardiac Arrest Care

Drug Therapy
IV/IO access
Epinephrine every 3-5 minutes
Amiodarone for refractory VF/VT

Consider Advanced Airway
Quantitative waveform capnography

Treat Reversible Causes

Continuous CPR

Monitor CPR Quality

© 2010 American Heart Association

CPR Quality
- Push hard (≥5 cm [2 inches]) and fast (≥100/min) and allow complete chest recoil
- Minimize interruptions in compressions
- Avoid excessive ventilation
- Rotate compressor every 2 minutes
- If no advanced airway, 30:2 compression-ventilation ratio
- Quantitative waveform capnography
  - If P_{ETCO_2} <10 mm Hg, attempt to improve CPR quality
- Intra-arterial pressure
  - If relaxation phase (diastolic) pressure <20 mm Hg, attempt to improve CPR quality

Return of Spontaneous Circulation (ROSC)
- Pulse and blood pressure
- Abrupt sustained increase in P_{ETCO_2} (typically ≥40 mm Hg)
- Spontaneous arterial pressure waves with intra-arterial monitoring

Shock Energy
- **Biphasic:** Manufacturer recommendation (e.g., initial dose of 120-200 J); if unknown, use maximum available. Second and subsequent doses should be equivalent, and higher doses may be considered.
- **Monophasic:** 360 J

Drug Therapy
- **Epinephrine IV/IO Dose:** 1 mg every 3-5 minutes
- **Vasopressin IV/IO Dose:** 40 units can replace first or second dose of epinephrine
- **Amiodarone IV/IO Dose:** First dose: 300 mg bolus. Second dose: 150 mg.

Advanced Airway
- Supraglottic advanced airway or endotracheal intubation
- Waveform capnography to confirm and monitor ET tube placement
- 8-10 breaths per minute with continuous chest compressions

Reversible Causes
- **H**ypovolemia
- **H**ypoxia
- **H**ydrogen ion (acidosis)
- **H**ypo-/hyperkalemia
- **H**ypothermia
- **T**ension pneumothorax
- **T**amponade, cardiac
- **T**oxins
- **T**hrombosis, pulmonary
- **T**hrombosis, coronary

Figure 28. The Cardiac Arrest Circular Algorithm.

Managing PEA: Diagnosing and Treating Underlying Causes

Introduction

Patients with PEA have poor outcomes. Rapid assessment and aggressive management offer the best chance of success. PEA may be caused by a reversible problem. If you can quickly identify a specific condition that has caused or is contributing to PEA and correct it, you may achieve ROSC. The identification of the underlying cause is of paramount importance in cases of PEA and asystole.

In the search for the underlying cause, do the following:

- Consider frequent causes of PEA by recalling the H's and T's
- Analyze the ECG for clues to the underlying cause
- Recognize hypovolemia
- Recognize drug overdose/poisonings

H's and T's

PEA is associated with many conditions. Healthcare providers should memorize the list of common causes to keep from overlooking an obvious cause of PEA that might be reversed by appropriate treatment.

The most common causes of PEA are presented as H's and T's in the table below:

H's	T's
Hypovolemia	**T**ension pneumothorax
Hypoxia	**T**amponade (cardiac)
Hydrogen ion (acidosis)	**T**oxins
Hyper-/hypokalemia	**T**hrombosis (pulmonary)
Hypothermia	**T**hrombosis (coronary)

Conditions and Management

The factors in the patient's history and physical exam that may help identify reversible causes of PEA have been combined with potentially effective interventions in Table 3.

Table 3. Potentially Reversible Causes of PEA and Asystole (H's and T's)

Condition	Clues From ECG and Monitor	Clues From History and Physical Examination	Potential Effective Interventions
Hypovolemia	Narrow complex Rapid rate	History, flat neck veins	Volume infusion
Hypoxia	Slow rate (hypoxia)	Cyanosis, blood gases, airway problems	Oxygenation, ventilation, advanced airway
Hydrogen ion (acidosis)	Smaller-amplitude QRS complexes	History of diabetes, bicarbonate-responsive preexisting acidosis, renal failure	Ventilation, sodium bicarbonate
Hyperkalemia *or*	*"High-potassium" ECG:* • T waves taller and peaked • P waves get smaller • QRS widens • Sine-wave PEA	History of renal failure, diabetes, recent dialysis, dialysis fistulas, medications	*Hyperkalemia:* • Calcium chloride • Sodium bicarbonate • Glucose plus insulin • Possibly albuterol
Hypokalemia	*"Low-potassium" ECG:* • T waves flatten • Prominent U waves • QRS widens • QT prolongs • Wide-complex tachycardia	Abnormal loss of potassium, diuretic use	*Hypokalemia:* • Add magnesium if cardiac arrest
Hypothermia	Osborne J waves	History of exposure to cold, central body temperature	See Hypothermia Algorithm (ECC Handbook)

(continued)

(continued)

Condition	Clues From ECG and Monitor	Clues From History and Physical Examination	Potential Effective Interventions
Tension pneumothorax	Narrow complex Slow rate (hypoxia)	History, no pulse felt with CPR, neck vein distention, tracheal deviation, unequal breath sounds, difficult to ventilate patient	Needle decompression Tube thoracostomy
Tamponade, cardiac	Narrow complex Rapid rate	History, no pulse felt with CPR, vein distention	Pericardiocentesis
Toxins (drug overdose): tricyclics, digoxin, β-blockers, calcium channel blockers	Various effects on ECG, predominately prolongation of QT interval	Bradycardia, empty bottles at the scene, pupils, neurologic exam	Intubation, specific antidotes and agents per toxidrome
Thrombosis, lungs: massive pulmonary embolism	Narrow complex Rapid rate	History, no pulse felt with CPR, distended neck veins, prior positive test for deep vein thrombosis or pulmonary embolism	Surgical embolectomy, fibrinolytics
Thrombosis, heart: acute, massive MI	Abnormal 12-lead ECG: • Q waves • ST-segment changes • T waves, inversions	History, cardiac markers, good pulse with CPR	

Analyze ECG for Clues to Underlying Cause

The ECG may provide valuable clues to the possible causes of PEA. Many providers think that the term *PEA* refers to the broad, slurred, slow, and disorganized electrical activity that bears no similarity to a normal P wave–QRS–T wave complex. The ECG, however, may display normal intervals or complexes or both. For example, sinus rhythm due to hypovolemia or sepsis may present as PEA. Other ECG findings in PEA may include wide-complex QRS.

Reassess the monitored rhythm and note the rate and width of the QRS complexes. PEA with narrow complexes is more likely to have a noncardiac cause.

Hypovolemia

Hypovolemia, a common cause of PEA, initially produces the classic physiologic response of a *rapid, narrow-complex tachycardia (sinus tachycardia)* and typically produces increased diastolic and decreased systolic pressures. As loss of blood volume continues, blood pressure drops, eventually becoming undetectable, but the narrow QRS complexes and rapid rate continue (i.e., PEA).

You should consider hypovolemia as a cause of hypotension, which can deteriorate to PEA. Providing prompt treatment can reverse the pulseless state by rapidly correcting the hypovolemia. Common nontraumatic causes of hypovolemia include occult internal hemorrhage and severe dehydration. Consider volume infusion for PEA associated with a narrow-complex tachycardia.

Cardiac and Pulmonary Conditions

ACS involving a large amount of heart muscle can present as PEA. That is, occlusion of the left main or proximal left anterior descending coronary artery can present with cardiogenic shock rapidly progressing to cardiac arrest and PEA. However, in patients with cardiac arrest and without known pulmonary embolism (PE), routine fibrinolytic treatment given during CPR shows no benefit and is not recommended.

Massive or saddle PE obstructs flow to the pulmonary vasculature and causes acute right heart failure. In patients with cardiac arrest due to presumed or known PE, it is reasonable to administer fibrinolytics.

Cardiac tamponade may be a reversible condition. Volume infusion in this condition may also help while definitive therapy is initiated. Tension pneumothorax can be effectively treated once recognized.

Note that cardiac tamponade, tension pneumothorax, and massive PE cannot be treated unless recognized. Bedside ultrasound, when performed by a skilled provider, may aid in rapid identification of tamponade and PE. There is growing evidence that pneumothorax can be identified using bedside ultrasound as well. Treatment for cardiac tamponade may require pericardiocentesis. Tension pneumothorax requires needle aspiration and chest tube placement. These procedures are beyond the scope of the ACLS Provider Course.

Drug Overdoses or Toxic Exposures

Certain drug overdoses and toxic exposures may lead to peripheral vascular dilatation and/or myocardial dysfunction with resultant hypotension. These are another cause of PEA. The approach to poisoned patients should be aggressive because the toxic effects may progress rapidly and may be of limited duration. In these situations myocardial dysfunction and arrhythmias may be reversible. Numerous case reports confirm the success of many specific limited interventions with one thing in common—they buy time.

Treatments that can provide this level of support include:

- Prolonged basic CPR in special resuscitation situations
- Cardiopulmonary bypass
- Intra-aortic balloon pumping
- Renal dialysis
- Specific drug antidotes (digoxin immune Fab, glucagon, bicarbonate)
- Transcutaneous pacing (TCP)
- Correction of severe electrolyte disturbances (potassium, magnesium, calcium, acidosis)
- Specific adjunctive agents (e.g., naloxone)

Remember, if the patient shows signs of ROSC, post–cardiac arrest care should be initiated.

Critical Concepts Common Reversible Causes of PEA	• Hypovolemia and hypoxia are the 2 most common and easily reversible causes of PEA. Be sure to look for evidence of these problems as you assess the patient.

Asystole Case

Introduction

In this case the *patient is in cardiac arrest.* Team members initiate and perform high-quality CPR throughout the BLS Survey and the ACLS Survey. The team interrupts CPR for 10 seconds or less for a rhythm check. *This patient has no pulse and the rhythm on the monitor is asystole.* Chest compressions resume immediately. The team leader now directs the team in the steps outlined in the asystole pathway of the Cardiac Arrest Algorithm (Figure 27, page 80), beginning with Box 10.

IV/IO access is a priority over advanced airway management unless bag-mask ventilation is ineffective or the arrest is caused by hypoxia. All resuscitation team members must simultaneously conduct a search for an underlying and treatable cause of the asystole in addition to performing their assigned roles.

At the end of this case the team will discuss the criteria for terminating resuscitative efforts; in some cases we must recognize that the patient is dead and that it would be more appropriate to direct efforts to supporting the family.

Learning Objectives

By the end of the case you should be able to:

1. Discuss when resuscitation should not be initiated, including do-not-attempt-resuscitation (DNAR) orders

2. Recall why survival from asystole is poor

3. Differentiate asystole and PEA: causes, treatments, and early, diligent search for correctable causes

4. Recall reversible causes of asystole

5. Outline treatments for causes of asystole

6. Describe the Cardiac Arrest Algorithm for asystole

7. Describe correct dosages and administration of epinephrine and vasopressin during cardiac arrest

8. Assign team member roles: monitor performance

Rhythms for Asystole

You will need to recognize the following rhythms:

- Asystole
- Slow PEA terminating in bradyasystolic rhythm

Drugs for Asystole

This case involves these drugs:

- Epinephrine
- Vasopressin

Approach to Asystole

Introduction

Asystole is a cardiac arrest rhythm associated with no discernible electrical activity on the ECG (also referred to as *flat line*). You should confirm that the flat line on the monitor is indeed "true asystole" by validating that the flat line is:

- Not another rhythm (e.g., fine VF) masquerading as a flat line
- Not the result of an operator error

Foundational Facts **Asystole and Technical Problems**	Asystole is a specific diagnosis, but flat line is not. The term *flat line* is nonspecific and can result from several possible conditions, including absence of cardiac electrical activity, lead or other equipment failure, and operator error. Some defibrillators and monitors signal the operator when a lead or other equipment failure occurs. Some of these problems are not applicable to all defibrillators.
	For a patient with cardiac arrest and asystole, quickly rule out any other causes of an isoelectric ECG, such as:
	• Loose leads or leads not connected to the patient or defibrillator/monitor • No power • Signal gain (amplitude/signal strength) too low

Patients With DNAR Orders

During the BLS Survey and ACLS Survey, you should be aware of reasons to stop or withhold resuscitative efforts. Some of these are:

- Rigor mortis
- Indicators of DNAR status (e.g., bracelet, anklet, written documentation)
- Threat to safety of providers

Out-of-hospital providers need to be aware of EMS-specific policies and protocols applicable to these situations. In-hospital providers and resuscitation teams should be aware of advance directives or specific limits to resuscitation attempts that are in place. That is, some patients may consent to CPR and defibrillation but not to intubation or invasive procedures. Many hospitals will record this in the medical record.

Asystole as an End Point

The prognosis for cardiac arrest with asystole is very poor. A large percentage of asystolic patients do not survive. Often asystole represents the final rhythm. Cardiac function has diminished until electrical and functional cardiac activity finally stop and the patient dies. Asystole is also the final rhythm of a patient initially in VF or VT.

Prolonged efforts are unnecessary and futile unless special resuscitation situations exist, such as hypothermia and drug overdose.

Managing Asystole

Overview

The management of asystole consists of the following components:

- Implementing the steps in the Cardiac Arrest Algorithm
- Identifying and correcting underlying causes
- Terminating efforts as appropriate

Cardiac Arrest Algorithm

As described in the VF/Pulseless VT and PEA Cases, the Cardiac Arrest Algorithm consists of 2 pathways (Figure 27). The left side of the algorithm outlines treatment for a shockable rhythm (VF/pulseless VT). The right side of the algorithm (Boxes 9 through 11) outlines treatment for a nonshockable rhythm (asystole/PEA). In both pathways therapies are designed around periods (2 minutes or 5 cycles) of uninterrupted, high-quality CPR. In this case we will focus on the asystole component of the asystole/PEA pathway.

Identification and Correction of Underlying Cause	Treatment of asystole is not limited to the interventions outlined in the algorithm. Healthcare providers should attempt to identify and correct an underlying cause if present. Rescuers must stop, think, and ask "Why did *this* person have *this* cardiac arrest at *this* time?" It is essential to search for and treat reversible causes of asystole for resuscitative efforts to be potentially successful. Use the H's and T's to recall conditions that could have contributed to asystole. See column on the right of the algorithm and the PEA case for more information on the H's and T's, including clinical clues and suggested treatments.

Application of the Cardiac Arrest Algorithm: Asystole Pathway

Introduction	In this case you have a patient in cardiac arrest. High-quality CPR is performed throughout the BLS Survey and the ACLS Survey. Interrupt CPR for 10 seconds or less while you perform a rhythm check. You interpret the rhythm on the monitor as asystole. CPR beginning with chest compressions for 2 minutes resumes immediately. You now conduct the steps outlined in the asystole pathway of the Cardiac Arrest Algorithm beginning with Box 9. At the same time you are searching for a possible underlying cause of the asystole.
Confirmed Asystole	Give priority to IV/IO access. Do not routinely insert an advanced airway unless ventilations with a bag-mask are ineffective. Do not interrupt CPR while establishing IV or IO access.

Administer Vasopressors (Box 10)	• Continue high-quality CPR, and as soon as IV/IO access is available, give a vasopressor as follows:

    – **Epinephrine** 1 mg IV/IO—repeat every 3 to 5 minutes

or

    – **Vasopressin** 40 units IV/IO to replace first or second dose of epinephrine

> *Administer drugs during CPR. Do not stop CPR to administer drugs.*

You can substitute vasopressin for either the first or second dose of epinephrine.

    • Consider advanced airway and capnography.

FYI 2010 Guidelines **No Atropine During Asystole**	• Although there is no evidence that atropine has detrimental effects during bradycardic or asystolic cardiac arrest, routine use of atropine during PEA or asystole is unlikely to have a therapeutic benefit. Atropine has been removed from the Cardiac Arrest Algorithm.

Decision Point: Rhythm Check	Check the rhythm after 2 minutes (about 5 cycles) of CPR.

> *Interruption of chest compressions to conduct a rhythm check should not exceed 10 seconds.*

Nonshockable Rhythm (Boxes 11 and 12)	• If *no electrical activity is present* (asystole), go back to Box 10 or 11. • If electrical activity is present, try to palpate a pulse. • If *no pulse is present* or if there is any doubt about the presence of a pulse, continue CPR, starting with chest compressions for 2 minutes. Go back to Box 10 and repeat the sequence. • If a *good pulse is present and the rhythm is organized,* begin post–cardiac arrest care.

Shockable Rhythm (Box 11)

If the rhythm check reveals a shockable rhythm, prepare to deliver a shock (resuming chest compressions during charging if appropriate). Refer to the left side of the algorithm and perform steps according to the VF/VT sequence, starting with Box 5 or 7.

Asystole and PEA Treatment Sequences

The diagram in Figure 28 (in the previous case, PEA) summarizes the recommended sequence of CPR, rhythm checks, and delivery of drugs for PEA and asystole based on expert consensus.

TCP Not Recommended

Several randomized controlled trials failed to show benefit from attempted TCP for asystole. At this time, the use of TCP is not recommended for patients with asystolic cardiac arrest.

Routine Shock Administration Not Recommended

There is no evidence that attempting to "defibrillate" asystole is beneficial. In one study the group that received shocks had a trend toward worse outcome. Given the importance of minimizing interruption of chest compressions, there is no justification for interrupting chest compressions to deliver a shock to patients with asystole.

When in Doubt

If it is unclear whether the rhythm is fine VF or asystole, an initial attempt at defibrillation may be warranted. Fine VF may be the result of a prolonged arrest. At this time the benefit of delaying defibrillation to perform CPR before defibrillation is unclear. EMS system medical directors may consider implementing a protocol that allows EMS responders to provide CPR while preparing for defibrillation of patients found by EMS personnel to be in VF.

Terminating Resuscitative Efforts

Terminating In-Hospital Resuscitative Efforts

If rescuers cannot rapidly identify a reversible cause and the patient fails to respond to the BLS and ACLS Surveys and subsequent interventions, termination of all resuscitative efforts should be considered.

The decision to terminate resuscitative efforts rests with the treating physician in the hospital and is based on consideration of many factors, including:

- Time from collapse to CPR
- Time from collapse to first defibrillation attempt
- Comorbid disease
- Prearrest state
- Initial arrest rhythm
- Response to resuscitative measures

None of these factors alone or in combination is clearly predictive of outcome. However, the duration of resuscitative efforts is an important factor associated with poor outcome. The chance that the patient will survive to hospital discharge and be neurologically intact diminishes as resuscitation time increases. Stop the resuscitation attempt when you determine with a high degree of certainty that the patient will not respond to further ACLS.

Terminating Out-of-Hospital Resuscitative Efforts

Continue out-of-hospital resuscitative efforts until one of the following occurs:

- Restoration of effective, spontaneous circulation and ventilation
- Transfer of care to a senior emergency medical professional
- The presence of reliable criteria indicating irreversible death
- The healthcare provider is unable to continue because of exhaustion or dangerous environmental hazards or because continued resuscitation places the lives of others in jeopardy
- A valid DNAR order is presented
- Online authorization from the medical control physician or by prior medical protocol for termination of resuscitation

Duration of Resuscitative Efforts

Available scientific studies demonstrate that in the absence of mitigating factors, prolonged resuscitative efforts are unlikely to be successful. The final decision to stop resuscitative efforts can never be as simple as an isolated time interval. If ROSC of any duration occurs, it may be appropriate to consider extending the resuscitative effort.

Experts have developed clinical rules to assist in decisions to terminate resuscitative efforts for in-hospital and out-of-hospital arrests. You should familiarize yourself with the established policy or protocols for your hospital or EMS system.

It may also be appropriate to consider other issues, such as drug overdose and severe prearrest hypothermia (e.g., submersion in icy water) when deciding whether to extend resuscitative efforts. Special resuscitation interventions and prolonged resuscitative efforts may be indicated for patients with hypothermia, drug overdose, or other potentially reversible causes of arrest.

Asystole: An Agonal Rhythm Confirming Death

You will see asystole most frequently in 2 situations:

- As a terminal rhythm in a resuscitation attempt that started with another rhythm
- As the first rhythm identified in a patient with unwitnessed or prolonged arrest

In either of these scenarios, asystole most often represents an agonal rhythm confirming death rather than a rhythm to be treated or a patient who can be resuscitated if the attempt persists long enough. Persistent asystole represents extensive myocardial ischemia and damage from prolonged periods of inadequate coronary perfusion. Prognosis is very poor unless a special resuscitation circumstance or immediately reversible cause is present. Survival from asystole is better for in-hospital than for out-of-hospital arrests according to data from Get With The Guidelines®–Resuscitation, formerly the National Registry of CPR.

Ethical Considerations

The resuscitation team must make a conscientious and competent effort to give patients "a trial of CPR and ACLS," provided the patient had not expressed a decision to forego resuscitative efforts and the victim is not obviously dead (e.g., rigor mortis, decomposition, hemisection, decapitation). The final decision to stop resuscitative efforts can never be as simple as an isolated time interval.

Transport of Patients in Cardiac Arrest

Emergency medical response systems should not require field personnel to transport every patient in cardiac arrest back to a hospital or to an ED. Transportation with continuing CPR is justified if interventions available in the ED cannot be performed in the out-of-hospital setting and they are indicated for special circumstances (i.e., cardiopulmonary bypass or extracorporeal circulation for patients with severe hypothermia).

After out-of-hospital cardiac arrest with ROSC, transport the patient to an appropriate hospital with a comprehensive post–cardiac arrest treatment system of care that includes acute coronary interventions, neurologic care, goal-directed critical care, and hypothermia. Transport the in-hospital post–cardiac arrest patient to an appropriate critical care unit capable of providing comprehensive post–cardiac arrest care.

Acute Coronary Syndromes Case

Introduction

The ACLS provider must have the basic knowledge to assess and stabilize patients with ACS. *Patients in this case have signs and symptoms of ACS, including possible AMI.* You will use the ACS Algorithm as the guide to clinical strategy.

The initial 12-lead ECG is used in all ACS cases to classify patients into 1 of 3 ECG categories, each with different strategies of care and management needs. These 3 ECG categories are ST-segment elevation suggesting current injury, ST-segment depression suggesting ischemia, and nondiagnostic or normal ECG. These are outlined in the ACS Algorithm, but STEMI with time-sensitive reperfusion strategies is the focus of this course (Figure 30).

Key components of this case are:

- Identification, assessment, and triage of acute ischemic chest discomfort
- Initial treatment of possible ACS
- Emphasis on early reperfusion of the patient with ACS/STEMI

Learning Objectives

By the end of this case you should be able to:

1. Discuss the differential diagnosis of life-threatening chest discomfort

2. Apply the ACS Algorithm for initial use of drugs

3. Apply the ACS Algorithm for initial drug doses

4. Apply the ACS Algorithm for initial resuscitation strategies and triage patients with sudden cardiac death to PCI facilities

5. Explain early identification of patients with ACS

6. Explain risk stratification of patients with ACS

7. Explain initial treatment of patients with ACS

8. Explain actions, indications, precautions, contraindications, dosage, and administration for oxygen, aspirin, nitroglycerin, morphine, and heparin (low-molecular-weight heparin [LMWH] or unfractionated heparin [UFH])

9. Describe guidelines for reperfusion strategies

Rhythms for ACS

Sudden cardiac death due to VF and hypotensive bradyarrythmias occurs with acute ischemia. Providers will understand to anticipate these rhythms and be prepared for immediate attempts at defibrillation and administration of drug or electrical therapy for symptomatic bradyarrhythmias.

Although 12-lead ECG interpretation is beyond the scope of the ACLS Provider Course, some ACLS providers will have 12-lead ECG reading skills. For them, this case summarizes the identification and management of patients with STEMI.

Drugs for ACS

Drug therapy and treatment strategies continue to evolve rapidly in the field of ACS. ACLS providers and instructors will need to monitor important changes. The ACLS Provider Course presents only basic knowledge focusing on early treatment and the priority of rapid reperfusion, relief of ischemic pain, and treatment of early life-threatening complications. Reperfusion may involve the use of fibrinolytic therapy or coronary angiography with PCI (i.e., balloon angioplasty/stenting). When used as the initial reperfusion strategy for STEMI, PCI is called *primary percutaneous coronary intervention* or PPCI.

Treatment of ACS involves the initial use of drugs to relieve ischemic discomfort, dissolve clots, and inhibit thrombin and platelets. These drugs are:

- Oxygen
- Aspirin
- Nitroglycerin
- Morphine
- Fibrinolytic therapy (overview)
- Heparin (UFH, LWMH)

Additional agents that are adjunctive to initial therapy and will not be discussed in the ACLS Provider Course are:

- β-Blockers
- Adenosine diphosphate (ADP) antagonists (clopidogrel, prasugrel)
- Angiotensin-converting enzyme (ACE) inhibitors
- HMG-CoA reductase inhibitor (statin therapy)

Goals for ACS Patients

Foundational Facts

Out-of-Hospital Cardiac Arrest Response

Half of the patients who die of ACS do so before reaching the hospital. VF or pulseless VT is the precipitating rhythm in most of these deaths. VF is most likely to develop during the first 4 hours after onset of symptoms.

Communities should develop programs to respond to out-of-hospital cardiac arrest. Such programs should focus on:

- Recognizing symptoms of ACS
- Activating the EMS system, with EMS advance notification of the receiving hospital
- Providing early CPR
- Providing early defibrillation with AEDs available through public access defibrillation programs and first responders
- Providing a coordinated system of care among the EMS system, the ED, and Cardiology

FYI 2010 Guidelines

Goals of Therapy for ACS

The *2010 Guidelines for CPR and ECC* combined the primary and secondary goals and considered all goals "primary goals."

The primary goals are:

- Identification of patients with STEMI and triage for early reperfusion therapy
- Relief of ischemic chest discomfort
- Prevention of MACE, such as death, nonfatal MI, and the need for urgent postinfarction revascularization
- Treatment of acute, life-threatening complications of ACS, such as VF/pulseless VT, symptomatic bradycardias, and unstable tachycardias

Reperfusion therapy opens an occluded coronary artery with either drugs or mechanical means. "Clot buster" drugs are called *fibrinolytics*, a more accurate term than *thrombolytics*. PCI, performed in the heart catheterization suite following coronary angiography, allows balloon dilation and/or stent placement for an occluded coronary artery. PCI performed as the initial reperfusion method is called *primary* PCI.

Pathophysiology of ACS

Patients with coronary atherosclerosis may develop a spectrum of clinical syndromes representing varying degrees of coronary artery occlusion. These syndromes include unstable angina (UA), NSTEMI, and STEMI. Sudden cardiac death may occur with each of these syndromes. Figure 29 illustrates the pathophysiology of ACS.

A Unstable plaque
B Plaque rupture
C Unstable angina
D Microemboli
E Occlusive thrombus

Early plaque formation

Significant plaque formation — A

Plaque rupture/thrombus — B C D

Unstable angina/NSTEMI

STEMI — E

Resolution/stable angina

Figure 29. Pathophysiology of ACS.

Acute Coronary Syndromes

1
Symptoms suggestive of ischemia or infarction

2
EMS assessment and care and hospital preparation:
• Monitor, support ABCs. Be prepared to provide CPR and defibrillation
• Administer aspirin and consider oxygen, nitroglycerin, and morphine if needed
• Obtain 12-lead ECG; if ST elevation:
  – Notify receiving hospital with transmission or interpretation; note time of onset and first medical contact
• Notified hospital should mobilize hospital resources to respond to STEMI
• If considering prehospital fibrinolysis, use fibrinolytic checklist

3
Concurrent ED assessment (<10 minutes)
• Check vital signs; evaluate oxygen saturation
• Establish IV access
• Perform brief, targeted history, physical exam
• Review/complete fibrinolytic checklist; check contraindications
• Obtain initial cardiac marker levels, initial electrolyte and coagulation studies
• Obtain portable chest x-ray (<30 minutes)

Immediate ED general treatment
• If O₂ sat <94%, start **oxygen** at 4 L/min, titrate
• **Aspirin** 160 to 325 mg (if not given by EMS)
• **Nitroglycerin** sublingual or spray
• **Morphine** IV if discomfort not relieved by nitroglycerin

4
ECG interpretation

5
ST elevation or new or presumably new LBBB; strongly suspicious for injury
ST-elevation MI (STEMI)

9
ST depression or dynamic T-wave inversion; strongly suspicious for ischemia
High-risk unstable angina/ non–ST-elevation MI (UA/NSTEMI)

13
Normal or nondiagnostic changes in ST segment or T wave
Low-/intermediate-risk ACS

6
• **Start adjunctive therapies** as indicated
• **Do not delay reperfusion**

7
Time from onset of symptoms ≤12 hours?

>12 hours

≤12 hours

10
Troponin elevated or high-risk patient
Consider early invasive strategy if:
• Refractory ischemic chest discomfort
• Recurrent/persistent ST deviation
• Ventricular tachycardia
• Hemodynamic instability
• Signs of heart failure

14
Consider admission to ED chest pain unit or to appropriate bed and follow:
• Serial cardiac markers (including troponin)
• Repeat ECG/continuous ST-segment monitoring
• Consider noninvasive diagnostic test

11
Start adjunctive treatments as indicated
• Nitroglycerin
• Heparin (UFH or LMWH)
• Consider: PO β-blockers
• Consider: Clopidogrel
• Consider: Glycoprotein IIb/IIIa inhibitor

15
Develops 1 or more:
• Clinical high-risk features
• Dynamic ECG changes consistent with ischemia
• Troponin elevated

Yes

8
Reperfusion goals:
Therapy defined by patient and center criteria
• **Door-to–balloon inflation (PCI) goal of 90 minutes**
• **Door-to-needle (fibrinolysis) goal of 30 minutes**

12
Admit to monitored bed
Assess risk status
Continue ASA, heparin, and other therapies as indicated
• ACE inhibitor/ARB
• HMG CoA reductase inhibitor (statin therapy)
Not at high risk: cardiology to risk stratify

16
Abnormal diagnostic noninvasive imaging or physiologic testing?

Yes

No

17
If no evidence of ischemia or infarction by testing, can discharge with follow-up

No

© 2010 American Heart Association

Only workin about 70% Pts

Figure 30. The Acute Coronary Syndromes Algorithm.

Managing ACS: The Acute Coronary Syndromes Algorithm

**Overview
of the Algorithm**

[handwritten margin notes:]
Anterior Wall:
- LV failure common
- Nitro Good

Inferior Wall
- Get 15 lead ECG
- Bradycardia
- Limited use Nitro

The Acute Coronary Syndromes Algorithm (Figure 30) outlines the assessment and management steps for a patient presenting with symptoms suggestive of ACS. The EMS responder in the out-of-hospital environment can begin immediate assessments and actions. These include giving oxygen, aspirin, nitroglycerin, and morphine if needed, and obtaining an initial 12-lead ECG (Box 2). Based on the ECG findings, the EMS provider may complete a fibrinolytic therapy checklist and notify the receiving ED of a potential AMI-STEMI when appropriate (Box 3). If out-of-hospital providers are unable to complete these initial steps before the patient's arrival at the hospital, the ED provider should implement this component of care.

Subsequent treatment occurs on the patient's arrival at the hospital. ED personnel should review the out-of-hospital 12-lead ECG if available. If not performed, acquisition of the 12-lead ECG should be a priority. The goal is to analyze the 12-lead ECG within 10 minutes of the patient's arrival in the ED (Box 4). Hospital personnel should categorize patients into 1 of 3 groups according to analysis of the ST segment or the presence of left bundle branch block (LBBB) on the 12-lead ECG. Treatment recommendations are specific to each group.

- STEMI
- High-risk UA/non–ST-elevation MI (NSTEMI)
- Intermediate/low-risk UA

The ACS Case will focus on the early reperfusion of the STEMI patient, emphasizing initial care and rapid triage for reperfusion therapy.

**Important
Considerations**

The ACS Algorithm (Figure 30) provides general guidelines that apply to the initial triage of patients based on symptoms and the 12-lead ECG. Healthcare personnel often obtain serial cardiac markers (cardiac troponins, CK-MB) in most patients that allow additional risk stratification and treatment recommendations. Two important points for STEMI need emphasis:

- The ECG is central to the initial risk and treatment stratification process.
- Healthcare personnel do not need evidence of elevated cardiac markers to make a decision to administer fibrinolytic therapy or perform diagnostic coronary angiography with coronary intervention (angioplasty/stenting) in STEMI patients.

**Application of the
ACS Algorithm**

The boxes in the algorithm guide assessment and treatment:

- Identification of chest discomfort suggestive of ischemia (Box 1)
- EMS assessment, care, transport, and hospital prearrival notification (Box 2)
- Immediate ED assessment and treatment (Box 3)
- Classification of patients according to ST-segment analysis (Boxes 5, 9, and 13)
- STEMI (Boxes 5 through 8)

FYI 2010 Guidelines

ACS Algorithm

- Changes to the ACS Algorithm were introduced to ensure prompt diagnosis and treatment. This offers the greatest potential benefit for myocardial salvage in the first hours of STEMI, and provides early and focused management of UA and NSTEMI. These changes should reduce adverse events and improve outcome.

Identification of Chest Discomfort Suggestive of Ischemia (Box 1)

Signs and Conditions   You should know how to identify chest discomfort suggestive of ischemia. Conduct a prompt and targeted evaluation of every patient whose initial complaints suggest possible ACS.

The most common symptom of myocardial ischemia and infarction is retrosternal chest discomfort. The patient may perceive this discomfort more as pressure or tightness than actual pain.

Symptoms suggestive of ACS may also include:

- Uncomfortable pressure, fullness, squeezing, or pain in the center of the chest lasting several minutes (usually more than a few minutes)
- Chest discomfort spreading to the shoulders, neck, one or both arms, or jaw
- Chest discomfort spreading into the back or between the shoulder blades
- Chest discomfort with light-headedness, dizziness, fainting, sweating, nausea, or vomiting
- Unexplained, sudden shortness of breath, which may occur with or without chest discomfort

Consider the likelihood that the presenting condition is ACS or one of its potentially lethal mimics. Other life-threatening conditions that may cause acute chest discomfort are aortic dissection, acute PE, acute pericardial effusion with tamponade, and tension pneumothorax.

Figure 31. The STEMI Chain of Survival.

Starting With Dispatch   All dispatchers and EMS providers must receive training in ACS symptom recognition along with the potential complications. Dispatchers, when authorized by medical control or protocol, should tell patients with no history of aspirin allergy or signs of active or recent gastrointestinal (GI) bleeding to chew an aspirin (160 to 325 mg) while waiting for EMS providers to arrive.

EMS Assessment, Care, and Hospital Preparation (Box 2)

Introduction   EMS assessment, care, and hospital preparation are outlined in Box 2. EMS responders may perform the following assessments and actions during the stabilization, triage, and transport of the patient to an appropriate facility:

- Monitor and support ABCs
- Administer aspirin and consider oxygen if O_2 saturation <94%, nitroglycerin, and morphine if discomfort unresponsive to nitrates
- Obtain a 12-lead ECG; interpret or transmit for interpretation
- Complete a fibrinolytic checklist if indicated
- Provide prearrival notification to the receiving facility if ST elevation

Monitor and Support ABCs

Monitoring and support of ABCs includes:

- Monitoring vital signs and cardiac rhythm
- Being prepared to provide CPR
- Using a defibrillator if needed

Administer Oxygen and Drugs

Providers should be familiar with the actions, indications, cautions, and treatment of side effects.

Oxygen

EMS providers should administer **oxygen** if the patient is dyspneic, is hypoxemic, has obvious signs of heart failure, has an arterial oxygen saturation <94% or the oxygen saturation is unknown. Providers should titrate oxygen therapy to a noninvasively monitored oxyhemoglobin saturation ≥94%. There is insufficient evidence to support the routine use of oxygen in uncomplicated ACS without signs of hypoxemia or heart failure or both.

Aspirin (Acetylsalicylic Acid)

If the patient has not taken **aspirin** and has no history of true aspirin allergy and no evidence of recent GI bleeding, give the patient aspirin (160 to 325 mg) to chew. In the initial hours of an ACS, aspirin is absorbed better when chewed than when swallowed, particularly if morphine has been given. Use rectal aspirin suppositories (300 mg) for patients with nausea, vomiting, active peptic ulcer disease, or other disorders of the upper GI tract.

Nitroglycerin (Glyceryl Trinitrate)

Give the patient 1 sublingual **nitroglycerin** tablet (or spray "dose") every 3 to 5 minutes for ongoing symptoms if it is permitted by medical control and no contraindications exist. Healthcare providers may repeat the dose twice (total of 3 doses). Administer nitroglycerin only if the patient remains hemodynamically stable: SBP is >90 mm Hg or no lower than 30 mm Hg below baseline (if known) and the heart rate is 50 to 100/min.

Nitroglycerin is a venodilator and needs to be used cautiously or not at all in patients with inadequate ventricular preload. These situations include:

- **Inferior wall MI and right ventricular (RV) infarction.** RV infarction may complicate an inferior wall MI. Patients with acute RV infarction are very dependent on RV filling pressures to maintain cardiac output and blood pressure. If RV infarction cannot be confirmed providers must use caution in administering nitrates to patients with inferior STEMI. If RV infarction is confirmed by right-sided precordial leads or clinical findings by an experienced provider, nitroglycerin and other vasodilators (morphine) or volume-depleting drugs (diuretics) are contraindicated as well.
- **Hypotension, bradycardia, or tachycardia.** Avoid use of nitroglycerin in patients with hypotension (SBP <90 mm Hg), marked bradycardia (<50/min), or tachycardia.
- **Recent phosphodiesterase inhibitor use.** Avoid the use of nitroglycerin if it is suspected or known that the patient has taken sildenafil or vardenafil within the previous 24 hours or tadalafil within 48 hours. Nitrates may cause severe hypotension refractory to vasopressor agents.

Morphine

Give **morphine** for chest discomfort unresponsive to sublingual or spray nitroglycerin if authorized by protocol or medical control. Morphine is indicated in STEMI when chest discomfort is unresponsive to nitrates. Use morphine with caution in UA/NSTEMI because of an association with increased mortality.

Morphine is an important treatment for ACS because it:

- Produces central nervous system analgesia, which reduces the adverse effects of neurohumoral activation, catecholamine release, and heightened myocardial oxygen demand
- Produces venodilation, which reduces left ventricular (LV) preload and oxygen requirements
- Decreases systemic vascular resistance, thereby reducing LV afterload
- Helps redistribute blood volume in patients with acute pulmonary edema

Remember, morphine is a venodilator. Like nitroglycerin, use morphine with caution in patients who may be preload dependent. If hypotension develops, administer fluids as a first line of therapy.

Critical Concepts Pain Relief With Nitroglycerin	• Relief of pain with nitroglycerin is neither specific nor a useful diagnostic tool to determine the etiology of symptoms in ED patients with chest pain or discomfort. GI etiologies as well as other causes of chest discomfort can "respond" to nitroglycerin administration. Therefore, the response to nitrate therapy is not diagnostic of ACS.

Caution Use of Nonsteroidal Anti-inflammatory Drugs	• Use of nonsteroidal anti-inflammatory drugs (NSAIDs) is contraindicated (except for aspirin) and should be discontinued. Both nonselective as well as COX-2 selective drugs should not be administered during hospitalization for STEMI because of the increased risk of mortality, reinfarction, hypertension, heart failure, and myocardial rupture associated with their use.

Obtain a 12-Lead ECG

EMS providers should obtain a 12-lead ECG. The *2010 Guidelines for CPR and ECC* recommends out-of-hospital 12-lead ECG diagnostic programs in urban and suburban EMS systems.

EMS Action	Recommendation
12-Lead ECG if available	HSFC recommends routine use of 12-lead out-of-hospital ECGs for patients with signs and symptoms of possible ACS.
Prearrival hospital notification for STEMI	Prearrival notification of the ED shortens the time to treatment (10 to 60 minutes has been achieved in clinical studies) and speeds reperfusion therapy with fibrinolytics or PCI or both, which may reduce mortality and minimize myocardial injury.
Fibrinolytic checklist if appropriate	If STEMI is identified on the 12-lead ECG, complete a fibrinolytic checklist if appropriate.

Immediate ED Assessment and Treatment (Box 3)

Introduction

The healthcare team should quickly evaluate the patient with potential ACS on the patient's arrival in the ED. Within the first 10 minutes, obtain a 12-lead ECG (if not already performed before arrival) and assess the patient.

> *The 12-lead ECG is at the center of the decision pathway in the management of ischemic chest discomfort and is the only means of identifying STEMI.*

A targeted evaluation should be performed and focus on chest discomfort, signs and symptoms of heart failure, cardiac history, risk factors for ACS, and historical features that may preclude the use of fibrinolytics. For the patient with STEMI, the goals of reperfusion are to give fibrinolytics within 30 minutes of arrival or perform PCI within 90 minutes of arrival.

Figure 32 shows how to measure ST-segment deviation.

Figure 32. How to measure ST-segment deviation. **A.** Inferior MI. The ST segment has no low point (it is coved or concave). **B.** Anterior MI.

Patient Assessment In <10 Minutes (Box 3)

Assessment of the patient in the first 10 minutes should include the following:

- Check vital signs and evaluate oxygen saturation.
- Establish IV access.
- Take a brief focused history and perform a physical examination.
- Complete the fibrinolytic checklist and check for contraindications, if indicated.
- Obtain a blood sample to evaluate initial cardiac marker levels, electrolytes, and coagulation.
- Obtain and review portable chest x-ray (<30 minutes after the patient's arrival in the ED). This should not delay fibrinolytic therapy for STEMI or activation of the PCI team for STEMI.

Note: The results of cardiac markers, chest x-ray, and laboratory studies should not delay reperfusion therapy unless clinically necessary, e.g., suspected aortic dissection or coagulopathy.

Patient General Treatment (Box 3)

Unless allergies or contraindications exist, 4 agents are routinely recommended for consideration in patients with ischemic-type chest discomfort:

- Oxygen if hypoxemic (O_2 % <94%) or signs of heart failure
- Aspirin
- Nitroglycerin
- Morphine (if ongoing discomfort or no response to nitrates)

Because these agents may have been given out of hospital, administer initial or supplemental doses as indicated. (See the discussion of these drugs in the previous section, "EMS Assessment, Care, and Hospital Preparation.")

Critical Concepts

Oxygen, Aspirin, Nitrates, Morphine

- Unless contraindicated, initial therapy with oxygen if needed, aspirin, nitrates, and, if indicated, morphine is recommended for all patients suspected of having ischemic chest discomfort.
- The major contraindication to nitroglycerin and morphine is hypotension, including hypotension from an RV infarction. The major contraindications to aspirin are true aspirin allergy and active or recent GI bleeding.

STEMI (Boxes 5 Through 8)

Introduction

Patients with STEMI usually have complete occlusion of an epicardial coronary artery.

> *The mainstay of treatment for STEMI is early reperfusion therapy achieved with fibrinolytics or primary PCI.*

Reperfusion therapy for STEMI is perhaps the most important advancement in treatment of cardiovascular disease in recent years. Early fibrinolytic therapy or direct catheter-based reperfusion has been established as a standard of care for patients with STEMI who present within 12 hours of onset of symptoms with no contraindications. Reperfusion therapy reduces mortality and saves heart muscle; the shorter the time to reperfusion, the greater the benefit. A 47% reduction in mortality was noted when fibrinolytic therapy was provided in the first hour after onset of symptoms.

Critical Concepts **Delay of Therapy**	• Routine consultation with a cardiologist or another physician should not delay diagnosis and treatment except in equivocal or uncertain cases. Consultation delays therapy and is associated with increased hospital mortality rates.
	• Potential delay during the in-hospital evaluation period may occur from **door** to data (ECG), from **data** to decision, and from **decision** to **drug** (or PCI). These 4 major points of in-hospital therapy are commonly referred to as the "4 D's."
	• All providers must focus on minimizing delays at each of these points. Out-of-hospital transport time constitutes only 5% of delay to treatment time; ED evaluation constitutes 25% to 33% of this delay.

Early Reperfusion Therapy

Rapidly identify patients with STEMI and quickly screen them for indications and contraindications to fibrinolytic therapy by using a fibrinolytic checklist if appropriate.

The first qualified physician who encounters a patient with STEMI should interpret or confirm the 12-lead ECG, determine the risk/benefit of reperfusion therapy, and direct administration of fibrinolytic therapy or activation of the PCI team. Early activation of PCI may occur with established protocols. The following time frames are recommended:

- If the patient meets the criteria for *fibrinolytic therapy,* an ED door-to-needle time (needle time is the beginning of infusion of a fibrinolytic agent) of 30 minutes is the medical system goal that is considered the longest time acceptable. Systems should strive to achieve the shortest time possible.
- For *PCI,* this goal for ED door–to–balloon inflation time is 90 minutes.
- Patients who are ineligible for *fibrinolytic therapy* should be considered for transfer to a PCI facility regardless of delay. The system should prepare for a door-to-departure time of 30 minutes when a transfer decision is made.

Adjunctive treatments may also be indicated.

Classify Patients According to ST-Segment Deviation (Boxes 5, 9, and 13)

Classify Into 3 Groups Based on ST-Segment Deviation

Review the initial 12-lead ECG (Box 4) and classify patients into 1 of the 3 following clinical groups (Boxes 5, 9, and 13):

General Group	Description
STEMI	ST elevation
High-risk UA/NSTEMI	ST depression or dynamic T-wave inversion
Intermediate/low-risk UA	Normal or nondiagnostic ECG

- *STEMI* is characterized by ST-segment elevation in 2 or more contiguous leads or new LBBB. Threshold values for ST-segment elevation consistent with STEMI are J-point elevation greater than 2 mm (0.2 mV) in leads V2 and V3* and 1 mm or more in all other leads or by new or presumed new LBBB.
*2.5 mm in men <40 years; 1.5 mm in all women.
- *High-risk UA/NSTEMI* is characterized by ischemic ST-segment depression ≥0.5 mm (0.05 mV) or dynamic T-wave inversion with pain or discomfort. Nonpersistent or transient ST elevation ≥0.5 mm for <20 minutes is also included in this category.
- *Intermediate or low-risk UA* is characterized by normal or nondiagnostic changes in the ST segment or T wave that are inconclusive and require further risk stratification. This classification includes patients with normal ECGs and those with ST-segment deviation in either direction of <0.5 mm (0.05 mV) or T-wave inversion ≤2 mm or 0.2 mV. Serial cardiac studies and functional testing are appropriate. Note that additional information (troponin) may place the patient into a higher risk classification after initial classification.

The ECG classification of ischemic syndromes is not meant to be exclusive. A small percentage of patients with normal ECGs may be found to have MI, for example. If the initial ECG is nondiagnostic and clinical circumstances indicate (e.g., ongoing chest discomfort), repeat the ECG.

Use of Fibrinolytic Therapy

A fibrinolytic agent or "clot buster" is administered to patients with J-point ST-segment elevation greater than 2 mm (0.2 mV) in leads V_2 and V_3 and 1 mm or more in all other leads or by new or presumed new LBBB (e.g., leads III, aVF; leads V_3, V_4; leads I and aVL) without contraindications. Fibrin-specific agents are effective in achieving normal flow in about 50% of patients given these drugs. Examples of fibrin-specific drugs are rtPA, reteplase, and tenecteplase. Streptokinase was the first fibrinolytic used widely, but it is not fibrin specific. It is still the most common agent used worldwide for acute STEMI reperfusion therapy.

Considerations for the use of fibrinolytic therapy are as follows:

- In the absence of contraindications and in the presence of a favorable risk-benefit ratio, fibrinolytic therapy is one option for reperfusion in patients with STEMI and *onset of symptoms within 12 hours of presentation* with qualifying ECG findings and if PCI is not available within 90 minutes of first medical contact.
- In the absence of contraindications, it is also reasonable to give fibrinolytics to patients with *onset of symptoms within the prior 12 hours* and ECG findings consistent with true posterior MI. Experienced providers will recognize this as a condition where ST-segment depression in the early precordial leads is equivalent to ST-segment elevation in others. When these changes are associated with other ECG findings, it is suggestive of a "STEMI" on the posterior wall of the heart.
- Fibrinolytics are generally not recommended for patients presenting *>12 hours after onset of symptoms*. But they may be considered if ischemic chest discomfort continues with persistent ST-segment elevation.
- Do not give fibrinolytics to patients who present *>24 hours after the onset of symptoms* or patients with ST-segment depression unless a true posterior MI is suspected.

Use of PCI

The most commonly used form of PCI is coronary intervention with stent placement. *Primary PCI* is used as an alternative to fibrinolytics. *Rescue PCI* is used early after fibrinolytics in patients who may have persistent occlusion of the infarct artery (failure to reperfuse with fibrinolytics), although this term has been recently replaced and included by the term *pharmacoinvasive strategy*. PCI has been shown to be superior to fibrinolysis in the combined end points of death, stroke, and reinfarction in many studies for patients presenting between 3 and 12 hours after onset. However, these results have been achieved in experienced medical settings with skilled providers (performing >75 PCIs per year) at a skilled PCI facility (performing >200 PCIs for STEMI with cardiac surgery capabilities).

Considerations for the use of PCI include the following:

- At the time of publication of the *2010 Guidelines for CPR and ECC*, percutaneous coronary intervention is the treatment of choice for the management of STEMI when it can be performed effectively with a door-to-balloon time of <90 minutes from first medical contact by a skilled provider at a skilled PCI facility.
- Primary PCI may also be offered to patients presenting to non-PCI centers if PCI can be initiated promptly within 90 minutes from EMS arrival–to-balloon time at the PCI-capable hospital. The TRANSFER AMI (Trial of Routine Angioplasty and Stenting After Fibrinolysis to Enhance Reperfusion in Acute Myocardial Infarction) trial supports the transfer of high-risk patients who receive fibrinolysis in a non-PCI center witihin 12 hours of symptom onset to a PCI center within 6 hours of fibrinolytic administration to receive routine early PCI.

- For patients admitted to a hospital without PCI capabilities, there may be some benefit associated with transfer for PCI versus administration of on-site fibrinolytics in terms of reinfarction, stroke, and a trend to lower mortality when PCI can be performed within 90 minutes of onset of STEMI.
- PCI is also preferred in patients with contraindications to fibrinolytics and is indicated in patients with cardiogenic shock or heart failure complicating MI.
- In patients with STEMI who present *3 hours or less from onset of symptoms*, treatment is more time sensitive, and PCI is superior to fibrinolysis.

Adjunctive Treatments

Other drugs are useful when indicated in addition to oxygen, sublingual or spray nitroglycerin, aspirin, morphine, and fibrinolytic therapy. These include:

- IV nitroglycerin
- Heparin
- Clopidogrel
- β-Blockers
- ACE inhibitors
- HMG–CoA reductase inhibitor therapy (statin)

IV nitroglycerin and heparin are commonly used early in the management of patients with STEMI. These agents are briefly discussed below. We will not review the use of β-blockers, ACE inhibitors, and statin therapy in STEMI. Use of these agents requires additional risk stratification skills and a detailed knowledge of the spectrum of ACS and, in some instances, continuing knowledge of the results of clinical trials.

IV Nitroglycerin

Routine use of IV nitroglycerin is not indicated and has not been shown to significantly reduce mortality in STEMI. IV nitroglycerin is indicated and used widely in ischemic syndromes. It is preferred over topical or long-acting forms because it can be titrated in a patient with potentially unstable hemodynamics and clinical condition. Indications for initiation of IV nitroglycerin in STEMI are:

- Recurrent or continuing chest discomfort unresponsive to sublingual or spray nitroglycerin
- Pulmonary edema complicating STEMI
- Hypertension complicating STEMI

Treatment goals using IV nitroglycerin are as follows:

Treatment Goal	Management
Relief of ischemic chest discomfort	• Titrate to effect • Keep SBP >90 mm Hg • Limit drop in SBP to 30 mm Hg below baseline in hypertensive patients
Improvement in pulmonary edema and hypertension	• Titrate to effect • Limit drop in SBP to 10% of baseline in normotensive patients • Limit drop in SBP to 30 mm Hg below baseline in hypertensive patients

Heparin

Heparin is routinely given as an adjunct for PCI and fibrinolytic therapy with fibrin-specific agents (rtPA, reteplase, tenecteplase). It is also indicated in other specific high-risk situations, such as LV mural thrombus, atrial fibrillation, and prophylaxis for pulmonary thromboembolism in patients with prolonged bed rest and heart failure complicating MI. If you use these drugs you must be familiar with dosing schedules for specific clinical strategies.

> *The inappropriate dosing and monitoring of heparin therapy has caused excess intracerebral bleeding and major hemorrhage in STEMI patients. Providers using heparin need to know the indications, dosing, and use in the specific ACS categories.*
>
> *The dosing, use, and duration have been derived from use in clinical trials. Specific patients may require dose modification. See the ECC Handbook for weight-based dosing guidelines, intervals of administration, and adjustment (if needed) in renal function.*

Bradycardia Case

Introduction

This case discusses assessment and management of a *patient with symptomatic bradycardia* (heart rate <50/min).

The cornerstones of managing bradycardia are to:

- Differentiate between signs and symptoms that are caused by the slow rate versus those that are unrelated
- Correctly diagnose the presence and type of AV block
- Use atropine as the drug intervention of first choice
- Decide when to start TCP
- Decide when to start epinephrine or dopamine to maintain heart rate and blood pressure
- Know when to call for expert consultation regarding complicated rhythm interpretation, drugs, or management decisions

In addition, you must know the techniques and cautions for using TCP.

Learning Objectives

By the end of this case you should be able to:

1. Recognize signs and symptoms of symptomatic bradycardia

2. Recognize causes of symptomatic bradycardia

3. State treatments for symptomatic bradycardia

4. Determine whether signs and symptoms are caused by bradycardia or another condition

5. Identify second- and third-degree AV blocks

6. Describe indications for TCP and doses of drugs used to treat bradycardia: atropine, dopamine, and epinephrine

Rhythms for Bradycardia

This case involves these ECG rhythms:

- Sinus bradycardia
- First-degree AV block
- Second-degree AV block
  - Type I (Wenckebach/Mobitz I)
  - Type II (Mobitz II)
- Third-degree AV block

You should know the major AV blocks because important treatment decisions are based on the type of block present (Figure 33). Complete AV block is generally the most important and clinically significant degree of block. Also, complete or third-degree AV block is the degree of block most likely to cause cardiovascular collapse and require immediate pacing. *Recognition of a symptomatic bradycardia due to AV block is a primary goal.* Recognition of the type of AV block is a secondary goal.

Figure 33. Examples of AV block. **A.** Sinus bradycardia with borderline first-degree AV block. **B.** Second-degree AV block type I. **C.** Second-degree AV block type II. **D.** Complete AV block with a ventricular escape pacemaker (wide QRS: 0.12 to 0.14 second). **E.** Third-degree AV block with a junctional escape pacemaker (narrow QRS: <0.12 second).

Drugs for Bradycardia

This case involves these drugs:

- Atropine
- Dopamine (infusion)
- Epinephrine (infusion)

Description of Bradycardia

Definitions

Definitions used in this case are as follows:

Term	Definition
Bradyarrhythmia or bradycardia*	Any rhythm disorder with a heart rate <60/min—e.g., third-degree AV block—or sinus bradycardia. When bradycardia is the cause of symptoms, the rate is generally <50/min.
Symptomatic bradyarrhythmia	Signs and symptoms due to the slow heart rate
*For the purposes of this case we will use the term *bradycardia* interchangeably with *bradyarrhythmia* unless specifically defined.	

Symptomatic Bradycardia

Sinus bradycardia may have multiple causes. Some are physiologic and require no assessment or therapy. For example, a well-trained athlete may have a heart rate in the range of 40 to 50/min or occasionally lower.

In contrast, some patients have heart rates in the normal sinus range, but these heart rates are inappropriate or insufficient for them. This is called a *functional* or *relative* bradycardia. For example, a heart rate of 70/min is too slow for a patient in cardiogenic or septic shock.

This case will focus on the patient with a bradycardia and heart rate <50/min. Key to the case management is the determination of symptoms or signs due to the decreased heart rate. A symptomatic bradycardia exists clinically when 3 criteria are present:

1. The heart rate is slow.
2. The patient has symptoms.
3. The symptoms are due to the slow heart rate.

Signs and Symptoms

You must perform a focused history and physical examination to identify the signs and symptoms of a bradycardia.

Symptoms include chest discomfort or pain, shortness of breath, decreased level of consciousness, weakness, fatigue, light-headedness, dizziness, and presyncope or syncope.

Signs include hypotension, drop in blood pressure on standing (orthostatic hypotension), diaphoresis, pulmonary congestion on physical examination or chest x-ray, frank congestive heart failure or pulmonary edema, and bradycardia-related (escape) frequent premature ventricular complexes or VT.

Managing Bradycardia: The Bradycardia Algorithm

Overview of the Algorithm

The Bradycardia Algorithm (Figure 34) outlines the steps for assessment and management of a patient presenting with symptomatic bradycardia with pulse. Implementation of this algorithm begins with the identification of bradycardia (Box 1); the heart rate is <50/min. First steps include the components of the BLS Survey and the ACLS Survey, such as supporting circulation and airway management, giving oxygen, monitoring the rhythm and vital signs, establishing IV access, and obtaining a 12-lead ECG if available (Box 2). In the differential diagnosis you determine if the patient has signs or symptoms of poor perfusion and if these are caused by the bradycardia (Box 3).

The primary decision point in the algorithm is the determination of adequate perfusion. If the patient has adequate perfusion, you observe and monitor (Box 4). If the patient has poor perfusion, you administer atropine (Box 5). If atropine is ineffective, prepare for TCP or consider dopamine or epinephrine infusion (Box 5). If indicated, you prepare for trans-venous pacing, search for and treat contributing causes, and seek expert consultation (Box 6).

The treatment sequence in the algorithm is determined by the severity of the patient's condition. You may need to implement multiple interventions simultaneously. If cardiac arrest develops, go to the Cardiac Arrest Algorithm.

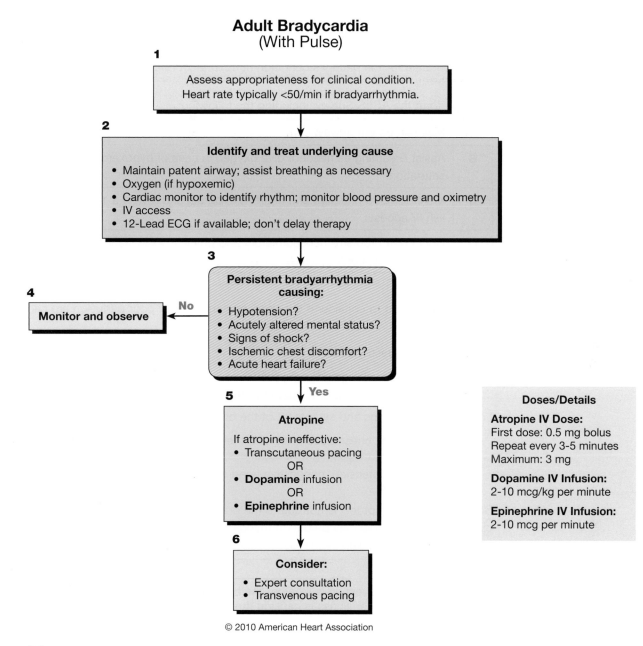

Figure 34. The Bradycardia Algorithm.

FYI 2010 Guidelines **The Bradycardia Algorithm**	• The Bradycardia Algorithm has been modified to reflect the changes in treatment presented in the *2010 Guidelines for CPR and ECC*. • The initial treatment of bradycardia is atropine. If bradycardia is unresponsive to atropine, IV infusion of β-adrenergic agonists with rate-accelerating effects (dopamine, epinephrine) or TCP can be effective while the patient is being prepared for emergent transvenous temporary pacing if required.

Application of the Bradycardia Algorithm

Introduction

In this case you have a patient presenting with symptoms of bradycardia. You conduct appropriate assessment and interventions as outlined in the Bradycardia Algorithm. At the same time you are searching for and treating possible contributing factors.

Identification of Bradycardia (Box 1)

Identify whether the bradycardia is:

- Present by definition, i.e., heart rate <50/min
- Inadequate for the patient's condition (functional or relative)

BLS and ACLS Surveys (Box 2)

Next, perform the ACLS Survey, including the following:

A	Maintain patent airway.
B	Assist breathing as needed; give oxygen in case of hypoxemia; monitor oxygen saturation.
C	Monitor blood pressure and heart rate; obtain and review a 12-lead ECG; establish IV access.
D	Conduct a problem-focused history and physical examination; search for and treat possible contributing factors.

Are Signs or Symptoms Caused by Bradycardia? (Box 3)

Box 3 prompts you to consider if the signs or symptoms of poor perfusion are caused by the bradycardia.

The key clinical questions are:

- Are there "serious" signs or symptoms?
- Are the signs and symptoms related to the slow heart rate?

Look for adverse signs and symptoms of the bradycardia:

- Symptoms (e.g., chest discomfort, shortness of breath, decreased level of consciousness, weakness, fatigue, light-headedness, dizziness, presyncope or syncope)
- Signs (e.g., hypotension, congestive heart failure, ventricular arrhythmias related to the bradycardia)

Sometimes the "symptom" is not due to the bradycardia. For example, hypotension associated with bradycardia may be due to myocardial dysfunction rather than the bradycardia. Keep this in mind when you reassess the patient's response to treatment.

Critical Concepts **Bradycardia**	• The key clinical question is whether the bradycardia is causing the patient's symptoms or some other illness is causing the bradycardia.

Decision Point: Adequate Perfusion?

You must now decide if the patient has adequate or poor perfusion.

- If the patient has **adequate perfusion,** observe and monitor (Box 4).
- If the patient has **poor perfusion,** proceed to Box 5.

Treatment Sequence Summary (Box 4)

If the patient has poor perfusion secondary to bradycardia, the treatment sequence is as follows:

Give atropine as first-line treatment		Atropine 0.5 mg IV—may repeat to a total dose of 3 mg
If atropine is ineffective		
Transcutaneous pacing	*or*	• Dopamine 2 to 10 mcg/kg per minute (chronotropic or heart rate dose) • Epinephrine 2 to 10 mcg/min

The treatment sequence is determined by the severity of the patient's clinical presentation. For patients with symptomatic bradycardia, move quickly through this sequence. These patients may be "pre–cardiac arrest" and may need multiple interventions simultaneously.

Treatment Sequence: Atropine

Any Symptomatic Bradycardia can recive atropine

In the absence of immediately reversible causes, atropine remains the first-line drug for acute symptomatic bradycardia. Atropine administration should not delay implementation of external pacing for patients with poor perfusion. Dopamine and epinephrine may be successful as an alternative to TCP.

For bradycardia, give atropine 0.5 mg IV every 3 to 5 minutes to a total dose of 0.04 mg/kg (maximum total dose of 3 mg). Atropine doses of <0.5 mg may paradoxically result in further slowing of the heart rate.

Use atropine cautiously in the presence of acute coronary ischemia or MI. An atropine-mediated increase in heart rate may worsen ischemia or increase infarct size.

Do not rely on atropine in Mobitz type II second- or third-degree AV block or in patients with third-degree AV block with a new wide QRS complex.

Treatment Sequence: Pacing

TCP may be useful for treatment of symptomatic bradycardia. TCP is noninvasive and can be performed by ACLS providers.

Healthcare providers should consider immediate pacing in unstable patients with high-degree heart block when IV access is not available. It is reasonable for healthcare providers to initiate TCP in unstable patients who do not respond to atropine.

Following initiation of pacing, confirm electrical and mechanical capture. Reassess the patient for symptom improvement and hemodynamic stability. Give analgesics and sedatives for pain control. Note that many of these drugs may further decrease blood pressure and affect the patient's mental status. Try to identify and correct the cause of the bradycardia.

Some limitations apply. TCP can be painful and may fail to produce effective electrical and mechanical capture. If symptoms are not caused by the bradycardia, pacing may be ineffective despite capture.

If you chose TCP as the second–line treatment and it is also ineffective (e.g., inconsistent capture), begin an infusion of dopamine or epinephrine and prepare for possible transvenous pacing by obtaining expert consultation.

Foundational Facts
Sedation and Pacing

Most conscious patients should be given sedation before pacing. If the patient is in cardiovascular collapse or rapidly deteriorating, it may be necessary to start pacing without prior sedation, particularly if drugs for sedation are not immediately available. The clinician must evaluate the need for sedation in light of the patient's condition and need for immediate pacing. A review of the drugs used is beyond the scope of the ACLS Provider Course. The general approach could include the following:

- Give parenteral benzodiazepine for anxiety and muscle contractions.
- Give a parenteral narcotic for analgesia.
- Use a chronotropic infusion once available.
- Obtain expert consultation for transvenous pacing.

Treatment Sequence: Epinephrine, Dopamine

Although β-adrenergic agonists with rate-accelerating effects are not first-line agents for treatment of symptomatic bradycardia, they are alternatives to TCP or in special circumstances such as overdose with a β-blocker or calcium channel blocker.

Because epinephrine and dopamine are vasoconstrictors, as well as chronotropes, healthcare providers must assess the patient's intravascular volume status and avoid hypovolemia when using these drugs.

Both epinephrine and dopamine infusions may be used for patients with symptomatic bradycardia, particularly if associated with hypotension, for whom atropine may be inappropriate or after atropine fails.

Begin epinephrine infusion at a dose of 2 to 10 mcg/min and titrate to patient response.

Begin dopamine infusion at 2 to 10 mcg/kg per minute and titrate to patient response. At lower doses dopamine has a more selective effect on inotropy and heart rate; at higher doses (>10 mcg/kg per minute) it also has vasoconstrictive effects.

Next Actions (Box 6)

After consideration of the treatment sequence in Box 5, you may need to:

- Prepare the patient for transvenous pacing
- Treat the contributing causes of the bradycardia
- Consider expert consultation—but do not delay treatment if the patient is unstable or potentially unstable

Transcutaneous Pacing

70-100mV enough to use get capture

Introduction

A variety of devices can pace the heart by delivering an electrical stimulus, causing electrical depolarization and subsequent cardiac contraction. TCP delivers pacing impulses to the heart through the skin by use of cutaneous electrodes. Most manufacturers have added a pacing mode to manual defibrillators.

The ability to perform TCP is now often as close as the nearest defibrillator. Providers need to know the indications, techniques, and hazards for using TCP.

Indications

Check femoral pulse after electrical capture

Indications for TCP are as follows:

- Hemodynamically unstable bradycardia (e.g., hypotension, acutely altered mental status, signs of shock, ischemic chest discomfort, acute heart failure hypotension)
- Unstable clinical condition likely due to the bradycardia
- For pacing readiness in the setting of AMI as follows:
  - Symptomatic sinus bradycardia
  - Mobitz type II second-degree AV block
  - Third-degree AV block
  - New left, right, or alternating bundle branch block or bifascicular block
- Bradycardia with symptomatic ventricular escape rhythms

Precautions

Precautions for TCP are as follows:

- TCP is contraindicated in severe hypothermia and is not recommended for asystole.
- Conscious patients require analgesia for discomfort unless delay for sedation will cause/contribute to deterioration.
- Do not assess the carotid pulse to confirm mechanical capture; electrical stimulation causes muscular jerking that may mimic the carotid pulse.

Technique

Perform TCP by following these steps:

Step	Action
1	Place pacing electrodes on the chest according to package instructions.
2	Turn the pacer ON.
3	Set the demand rate to approximately 60/min. This rate can be adjusted up or down (based on patient clinical response) once pacing is established.
4	Set the current milliamperes output 2 mA above the dose at which consistent capture is observed (safety margin).

External pacemakers have either *fixed* rates (asynchronous mode) or *demand* rates.

Assess Response to Treatment

Rather than target a precise heart rate, the goal of therapy is to ensure improvement in clinical status (i.e., signs and symptoms related to the bradycardia). Signs of hemodynamic impairment include hypotension, acutely altered mental status, signs of shock, ischemic chest discomfort, acute heart failure, or other signs of shock related to the bradycardia. Start pacing at a rate of about 60/min. Once pacing is initiated, adjust the rate based on the patient's clinical response. Most patients will improve with a rate of 60 to 70/min if the symptoms are primarily due to the bradycardia.

Consider giving atropine before pacing in mildly symptomatic patients. Do not delay pacing for unstable patients, particularly those with high-degree AV block. Atropine may increase heart rate, improve hemodynamics, and eliminate the need for pacing. If atropine is ineffective or likely to be ineffective or if establishment of IV access or atropine administration is delayed, begin pacing as soon as it is available.

Patients with ACS should be paced at the lowest heart rate that allows clinical stability. Higher heart rates can worsen ischemia because heart rate is a major determinate of myocardial oxygen demand. Ischemia, in turn, can precipitate arrhythmias.

An alternative to pacing if symptomatic bradycardia is unresponsive to atropine is a chronotropic drug infusion to stimulate heart rate:

- Epinephrine: Initiate at 2 to 10 mcg/min and titrate to patient response
- Dopamine: Initiate at 2 to 10 mcg/kg per minute and titrate to patient response

Bradycardia With Escape Rhythms

A bradycardia may lead to bradycardia-dependent ventricular rhythms. When the heart rate falls, an electrically unstable ventricular area may "escape" suppression by higher and faster pacemakers (e.g., sinus node), especially in the setting of acute ischemia. These ventricular rhythms often fail to respond to drugs. With severe bradycardia some patients will develop wide-complex ventricular beats that can precipitate VT or VF. Pacing may increase the heart rate and eliminate bradycardia-dependent ventricular rhythms. However, an accelerated idioventricular rhythm (sometimes called AIVR) may occur in the setting of inferior wall MI. This rhythm is usually stable and does not require pacing.

Patients with ventricular escape rhythms may have normal myocardium with disturbed conduction. After correction of electrolyte abnormalities or acidosis, rapid pacing can stimulate effective myocardial contractions until the conduction system recovers.

Standby Pacing

Several bradycardic rhythms in ACS are caused by acute ischemia of conduction tissue and pacing centers. Patients who are clinically stable may decompensate suddenly or become unstable over minutes to hours from worsening conduction abnormalities. These bradycardias may deteriorate to complete AV block and cardiovascular collapse.

Place or have ready TCP electrodes in anticipation of clinical deterioration in patients with acute myocardial ischemia or infarction associated with the following rhythms:

- Symptomatic sinus node dysfunction with severe and symptomatic sinus bradycardia
- Asymptomatic Mobitz type II second-degree AV block
- Asymptomatic third-degree AV block
- Newly acquired left, right, or alternating bundle branch block or bifascicular block in the setting of AMI

Unstable Tachycardia Case

Introduction

If you are the team leader in this case, you will conduct the assessment and management of a *patient with a rapid, unstable heart rate*. You must be able to classify the tachycardia and implement appropriate interventions as outlined in the Tachycardia Algorithm. You will be evaluated on your knowledge of the factors involved in safe and effective synchronized cardioversion as well as your performance of the procedure.

Learning Objectives

By the end of this case you should be able to:

1. Differentiate characteristics of stable and unstable tachycardias

2. Describe the ACLS priorities of care in the Tachycardia Algorithm

3. Identify unstable patients and follow this arm of the Tachycardia Algorithm

4. Describe energy levels required for electrical cardioversion of tachycardia varieties

5. Demonstrate safety procedures when performing cardioversion

Rhythms for Unstable Tachycardia

This case involves these ECG rhythms:

- Atrial fibrillation
- Atrial flutter
- Reentry supraventricular tachycardia (SVT)
- Monomorphic VT
- Polymorphic VT
- Wide-complex tachycardia of uncertain type

Drugs for Unstable Tachycardia

Drugs are generally not used to manage patients with unstable tachycardia. Immediate cardioversion is recommended. Consider administering sedative drugs in the conscious patient. But do not delay immediate cardioversion in the unstable patient.

The Approach to Unstable Tachycardia

Introduction

A tachyarrhythmia (rhythm with heart rate >100/min) has many potential causes and may be symptomatic or asymptomatic. The key to management of a patient with any tachycardia is to determine whether pulses are present. If pulses are present, determine whether the patient is stable or unstable and then provide treatment based on patient condition and rhythm.

If the tachyarrhythmia is sinus tachycardia, conduct a diligent search for the cause of the tachycardia. Treatment and correction of this cause will improve the signs and symptoms.

Definitions

Definitions used in this case are as follows:

Term	Definition
Tachyarrhythmia, tachycardia*	Heart rate >100/min
Symptomatic tachyarrhythmia	Signs and symptoms due to the rapid heart rate

*For the purposes of this case we will use the term *tachycardia* interchangeably with *tachyarrhthmia*. Sinus tachycardia will be specifically indicated.

Pathophysiology of Unstable Tachycardia

Unstable tachycardia exists when the heart rate is too fast for the patient's clinical condition and the excessive heart rate causes symptoms or an unstable condition because the heart is:

- *Beating so fast* that cardiac output is reduced; this can cause pulmonary edema, coronary ischemia, and reduced blood flow to vital organs (e.g., brain, kidneys)
- *Beating ineffectively* so that coordination between the atrium and ventricles or the ventricles themselves reduces cardiac output

Symptoms and Signs

Unstable tachycardia leads to serious signs and symptoms that include:

- Hypotension
- Acutely altered mental status
- Signs of shock
- Ischemic chest discomfort
- Acute heart failure (AHF)

Rapid Recognition Is the Key to Management

The 2 keys to management of patients with unstable tachycardia are:

1. Rapid recognition that the patient is *significantly symptomatic* or even *unstable*

2. Rapid recognition that the *signs and symptoms are caused by the tachycardia*

> *You must quickly determine whether the patient's tachycardia is producing hemodynamic instability and serious signs and symptoms or whether the signs and symptoms (e.g., the pain and distress of an AMI) are producing the tachycardia.*
>
> This determination can be difficult. Many experts suggest that when a heart rate is <150/min, it is unlikely that symptoms of instability are caused primarily by the tachycardia unless there is impaired ventricular function. A heart rate >150/min is an inappropriate response to physiologic stress (e.g., fever, dehydration) or other underlying conditions.

Severity

Assess for the presence or absence of signs and symptoms and for their severity. Frequent patient assessment is indicated.

Indications for Cardioversion

Rapid identification of symptomatic tachycardia will help you determine whether you should prepare for immediate cardioversion. For example:

- *Sinus tachycardia* is a physiologic response to extrinsic factors, such as fever, anemia, or hypotension/shock, which create the need for increased cardiac output. There is usually a high degree of sympathetic tone and neurohormonal factors. Sinus tachycardia will not respond to cardioversion. In fact, if a shock is delivered, the heart rate often increases.
- If the patient with tachycardia is stable (i.e., no serious signs related to the tachycardia), patients may await expert consultation because treatment has the potential for harm.
- *Atrial flutter* typically produces a heart rate of approximately 150/min (lower rates may be present in patients who have received antiarrhythmic therapy). Atrial flutter at this rate is often stable in the patient without heart or serious systemic disease.
- At rates >150/min, symptoms are often present and cardioversion is often required if the patient is unstable.
- If the patient is seriously ill or has underlying cardiovascular disease, symptoms may be present at lower rates.

You must know when cardioversion is indicated, how to prepare the patient for it (including appropriate medication), and how to switch the defibrillator/monitor to operate as a cardioverter.

Managing Unstable Tachycardia: The Tachycardia Algorithm

Introduction

The Tachycardia Algorithm simplifies initial management of tachycardia. The presence or absence of pulses is considered key to management of a patient with any tachycardia. If pulses are present, determine whether the patient is stable or unstable and then provide treatment based on the patient's condition and rhythm. If a pulseless tachycardia is present, then manage the patient according to the Cardiac Arrest Algorithm (Figure 19, page 61).

The ACLS provider should either be an expert or be able to obtain expert consultation. Actions in the boxes require advanced knowledge of ECG rhythm interpretation and antiarrhythmic therapy and are intended to be accomplished in the in-hospital setting with expert consultation available.

Overview

The Tachycardia Algorithm (Figure 35) outlines the steps for assessment and management of a patient presenting with symptomatic tachycardia with pulses. Implementation of this algorithm begins with the identification of tachycardia with pulses (Box 1). If a tachycardia and a pulse are present, perform assessment and management steps guided by the BLS Survey and the ACLS Survey (Box 2). The key in this assessment is to decide if the tachycardia is stable or unstable.

If signs and symptoms persist despite provision of supplementary oxygen and support of airway and circulation and if significant signs or symptoms are due to the tachycardia (Box 3), then the tachycardia is unstable and immediate synchronized cardioversion is indicated (Box 4).

If the patient is stable, you will evaluate the ECG, and determine if the QRS complex is wide or narrow and regular or irregular (Box 5). The treatment of stable tachycardia is presented in the next case (Box 6).

A precise diagnosis of the rhythm (e.g., reentry SVT, atrial flutter) may not be possible at this time.

| **Foundational Facts**

Serious or Significant Symptoms

Unstable Condition | Intervention is determined by the presence of significant symptoms or by an unstable condition resulting from the tachycardia.*

Serious symptoms and signs include:

• Hypotension
• Acutely altered mental status
• Signs of shock
• Ischemic chest discomfort
• Acute heart failure (AHF)

Ventricular rates <150/min usually do not cause serious signs or symptoms. |

| **FYI 2010 Guidelines**

Tachycardia With a Pulse Algorithm | • The 2010 Tachycardia With a Pulse Algorithm (Figure 35) is presented in the traditional box-and-line format. Overall, the algorithm has been simplified and redesigned to facilitate learning and memorization of the treatment recommendations and to emphasize the importance of identifying whether the tachycardia is a cause or a symptom of an underlying condition, which is fundamental to the management of all tachyarrhythmias. |

Summary

Your assessment and management of this patient will be guided by the following key questions presented in the Tachycardia Algorithm:

• Are symptoms present or absent?
• Is the patient stable or unstable?
• Is the QRS narrow or wide?
• Is the rhythm regular or irregular?
• Is the QRS monomorphic or polymorphic?

Your answers to these questions will determine the next appropriate steps.

Adult Tachycardia
(With Pulse)

1

Assess appropriateness for clinical condition.
Heart rate typically ≥150/min if tachyarrhythmia.

2

Identify and treat underlying cause

- Maintain patent airway; assist breathing as necessary
- Oxygen (if hypoxemic)
- Cardiac monitor to identify rhythm; monitor blood pressure and oximetry

3

Persistent tachyarrhythmia causing:

- Hypotension?
- Acutely altered mental status?
- Signs of shock?
- Ischemic chest discomfort?
- Acute heart failure?

Yes →

4

Synchronized cardioversion
- Consider sedation
- If regular narrow complex, consider adenosine

5

Wide QRS?
≥0.12 second

No ↓

Yes →

6

- IV access and 12-lead ECG if available
- Consider adenosine only if regular and monomorphic
- Consider antiarrhythmic infusion
- Consider expert consultation

No ↓

7

- IV access and 12-lead ECG if available
- Vagal maneuvers
- Adenosine (if regular)
- β-Blocker or calcium channel blocker
- Consider expert consultation

Doses/Details

Synchronized Cardioversion
Initial recommended doses:
- Narrow regular: 50-100 J
- Narrow irregular: 120-200 J biphasic or 200 J monophasic
- Wide regular: 100 J
- Wide irregular: defibrillation dose (NOT synchronized)

Adenosine IV Dose:
First dose: 6 mg rapid IV push; follow with NS flush.
Second dose: 12 mg if required.

Antiarrhythmic Infusions for Stable Wide-QRS Tachycardia

Procainamide IV Dose:
20-50 mg/min until arrhythmia suppressed, hypotension ensues, QRS duration increases >50%, or maximum dose 17 mg/kg given. Maintenance infusion: 1-4 mg/min. Avoid if prolonged QT or CHF.

Amiodarone IV Dose:
First dose: 150 mg over 10 minutes. Repeat as needed if VT recurs. Follow by maintenance infusion of 1 mg/min for first 6 hours.

Sotalol (not available in Canada) IV Dose:
100 mg (1.5 mg/kg) over 5 minutes. Avoid if prolonged QT.

© 2010 American Heart Association

Figure 35. The Tachycardia With a Pulse Algorithm.

Application of the Tachycardia Algorithm to the Unstable Patient

Introduction

In this case you have a patient with tachycardia and a pulse. You conduct the steps outlined in the Tachycardia Algorithm to evaluate and manage the patient.

Assess Appropriateness for Clinical Condition (Box 1)

- Tachycardia is defined as an arrhythmia with a rate >100/min.
- The rate takes on clinical significance at its greater extremes and is more likely attributable to an arrhythmia rate of ≥150/min.
- It is unlikely that symptoms of instability are caused primarily by the tachycardia when the heart rate is <150/min unless there is impaired ventricular function.

Confirm SVT vs VT w̄ 12 lead ECG

A Fib convert 120-200J if unstable

Identify and Treat the Underlying Cause: BLS and ACLS Surveys (Box 2)

Use the BLS Survey and the ACLS Survey to guide your approach.

- Look for signs of increased work of breathing (tachypnea, intercostal retractions, suprasternal retractions, paradoxical abdominal breathing) and hypoxemia as determined by pulse oximetry.
- Give oxygen, if indicated and monitor oxygen saturation.
- Obtain an ECG to identify the rhythm.
- Evaluate blood pressure.
- Establish IV access.
- Identify and treat reversible causes.

If symptoms persist despite support of adequate oxygenation and ventilation, proceed to Box 3.

Critical Concepts **Unstable Patients**	<ul><li>Healthcare providers should obtain a 12-lead ECG early in the assessment to better define the rhythm.</li><li>However, unstable patients require immediate cardioversion.</li><li>Do not delay immediate cardioversion for acquisition of the 12-lead ECG if the patient is unstable.</li></ul>

Decision Point: Is the Persistent Tachyarrhythmia Causing Significant Signs or Symptoms? (Box 3)

Assess the patient's degree of instability and determine if the instability is related to the tachycardia.

Unstable

If the patient demonstrates rate-related cardiovascular compromise with signs and symptoms such as hypotension, acutely altered mental status, signs of shock, ischemic chest discomfort, acute heart failure, or other signs of shock suspected to be due to a tachyarrhythmia, proceed to immediate synchronized cardioversion (Box 4).

Serious signs and symptoms are unlikely if the ventricular rate is <150/min in patients with a healthy heart. However, if the patient is seriously ill or has significant underlying heart disease or other conditions, symptoms may be present at a lower heart rate.

Stable

If the patient does not have rate-related cardiovascular compromise, proceed to Box 5. The healthcare provider has time to obtain a 12-lead ECG, evaluate the rhythm, determine if the width of the QRS, and determine treatment options. Stable patients may await expert consultation because treatment has the potential for harm.

Foundational Facts
Treatment Based on Type of Tachycardia

You may not always be able to distinguish between supraventricular and ventricular rhythms. Most wide-complex (broad-complex) tachycardias are ventricular in origin (especially if the patient has underlying heart disease or is older). If the patient is pulseless, treat the rhythm as VF and follow the Cardiac Arrest Algorithm.

If the patient has a wide-complex tachycardia and is unstable, assume it is VT until proven otherwise. The amount of energy required for cardioversion of VT is determined by the morphologic characteristics.

- If the patient is unstable but has a pulse with regular uniform wide-complex VT (*monomorphic VT*).
  - Treat with synchronized cardioversion and an initial shock of 100 J (monophasic waveform).
  - If there is no response to the first shock, increasing the dose in a stepwise fashion is reasonable.*
- Arrhythmias with a polymorphic QRS appearance (*polymorphic VT*), such as torsades de pointes will usually not permit synchronization. If the patient has *polymorphic VT*:
  - Treat as VF with high-energy unsynchronized shocks (e.g., defibrillation doses).

If there is any doubt about whether an unstable patient has monomorphic or polymorphic VT, do not delay treatment for further rhythm analysis. Provide high-energy, unsynchronized shocks.

*No studies that addressed this issue had been identified at the time that the manuscript for the *2010 Guidelines for CPR and ECC* was in preparation. Thus, this recommendation represents expert opinion.

Perform Immediate Synchronized Cardioversion (Box 4)

- If possible establish IV access before cardioversion and administer sedation if the patient is conscious.
- Do not delay cardioversion if the patient is extremely unstable.

Further information about cardioversion appears below.

If the patient with a regular narrow-complex SVT or a monomorphic wide-complex tachycardia is not hypotensive, healthcare providers may administer adenosine while preparing for synchronized cardioversion.

If cardiac arrest develops, see the Cardiac Arrest Algorithm.

Determine the Width of the QRS Complex (Box 5)

- If the width of the QRS complex is ≥0.12 second, go to Box 6.
- If the width of the QRS complex is <0.12 second, go to Box 7.

Cardioversion

Introduction

You must know when cardioversion is indicated and what type of shock to administer. Before cardioversion, establish IV access and sedate the responsive patient if possible, but do not delay cardioversion in the unstable or deteriorating patient.

This section discusses the following important concepts about cardioversion:

- The difference between unsynchronized and synchronized shocks
- Potential challenges to delivery of synchronized shocks
- Energy doses for specific rhythms

Unsynchronized vs Synchronized Shocks

Modern defibrillator/cardioverters are capable of delivering 2 types of shocks:

- Unsynchronized shocks
- Synchronized shocks

An *unsynchronized* shock simply means that the electrical shock will be delivered as soon as the operator pushes the SHOCK button to discharge the device. Thus, the shock may fall randomly anywhere within the cardiac cycle. *These shocks should use higher energy levels than synchronized cardioversion.*

Synchronized cardioversion uses a sensor to deliver a shock that is synchronized with a peak of the QRS complex (e.g., the highest point of the R wave). When this option (the "sync" option) is engaged, the operator presses the SHOCK button to deliver a shock. There will likely be a delay before the defibrillator/cardioverter delivers a shock because the device will synchronize shock delivery with the peak of the R wave in the patient's QRS complex. This synchronization may require analysis of several complexes. Synchronization avoids the delivery of a shock during cardiac repolarization (represented on the surface ECG as the T wave), a period of vulnerability in which a shock can precipitate VF. Synchronized cardioversion uses a lower energy level than attempted defibrillation. Low-energy shocks should always be delivered as synchronized shocks to avoid precipitating VF.

Potential Problems With Synchronization

In theory, synchronization is simple. The operator pushes the SYNC control on the face of the defibrillator/cardioverter. In practice, however, there are potential problems. For example:

- If the R-wave peaks of a tachycardia are undifferentiated or of low amplitude, the monitor sensors may be unable to identify an R-wave peak and therefore will not deliver the shock.
- Many cardioverters will not synchronize through the handheld quick-look paddles. An unwary practitioner may try to synchronize—unsuccessfully in that the machine will not discharge—and may not recognize the problem.
- Synchronization can take extra time (e.g., if it is necessary to attach electrodes or if the operator is unfamiliar with the equipment).

Recommendations

When to Use Synchronized Shocks

Synchronized shocks are recommended for patients with:

- Unstable SVT
- Unstable atrial fibrillation
- Unstable atrial flutter
- Unstable regular monomorphic tachycardia with pulses

When to Use Unsynchronized Shocks

Unsynchronized high-energy shocks are recommended:

- For a patient who is pulseless
- For a patient demonstrating clinical deterioration (in prearrest), such as those with severe shock or polymorphic VT, when you think a delay in converting the rhythm will result in cardiac arrest
- When you are unsure whether monomorphic or polymorphic VT is present in the unstable patient

Should the unsynchronized shock cause VF (occurring in only a very small minority of patients despite the theoretical risk), immediately attempt defibrillation.

Energy Doses for Cardioversion

Select the energy dose for the specific type of rhythm.

For unstable atrial fibrillation:

- Monophasic cardioversion: Deliver an initial 200-J synchronized shock.
- Biphasic cardioversion: Deliver an initial 120- to 200-J synchronized shock.
- In either case, increase the energy dose in a stepwise fashion for any subsequent cardioversion attempts.

A dose of 120 J to 200 J is reasonable with a biphasic waveform. Escalate the second and subsequent shock dose as needed.

Cardioversion of atrial flutter and SVT generally require less energy. An initial energy dose of 50 J to 100 J with a biphasic waveform is often sufficient. If the initial 50-J dose fails, increase the dose in a stepwise fashion.

Monomorphic VT (regular form and rate) with a pulse responds well to monophasic or biphasic waveform cardioversion (synchronized) shocks at an initial dose of 100 J. If there is no response to the first shock, increase the dose in a stepwise fashion. No studies were identified that addressed this issue. Thus, this recommendation represents expert opinion.

Synchronized Cardioversion Technique

Introduction

Synchronized cardioversion is the treatment of choice when a patient has a symptomatic (unstable) reentry SVT or VT with pulses. It is also recommended to treat unstable atrial fibrillation and unstable atrial flutter.

Cardioversion is unlikely to be effective for treatment of junctional tachycardia or ectopic or multifocal atrial tachycardia because these rhythms have an automatic focus arising from cells that are spontaneously depolarizing at a rapid rate. Delivery of a shock generally cannot stop these rhythms and may actually increase the rate of the tachyarrhythmia.

In synchronized cardioversion, shocks are administered through adhesive electrodes or handheld paddles. *You will need to place the defibrillator/monitor in synchronized (sync) mode.* The sync mode is designed to deliver energy just after the R wave of the QRS complex.

Technique

Follow these steps to perform synchronized cardioversion. Modify the steps for your specific device.

Step	Action
1	Sedate all conscious patients unless unstable or deteriorating rapidly.
2	Turn on the defibrillator (monophasic or biphasic).
3	Attach monitor leads to the patient ("white to right, red to ribs, what's left over to the left shoulder") and ensure proper display of the patient's rhythm. Position adhesive electrode (conductor) pads on the patient.
4	Press the SYNC control button to engage the synchronization mode.
5	Look for markers on the R wave indicating sync mode.
6	Adjust monitor gain if necessary until sync markers occur with each R wave.
7	Select the appropriate energy level. Deliver monophasic synchronized shocks in the following sequence: <table><tr><th>If</th><th>Initial Dose*</th></tr><tr><td>Unstable atrial fibrillation</td><td>200 J</td></tr><tr><td>Unstable monomorphic VT</td><td>100 J</td></tr><tr><td>Other unstable SVT Atrial flutter</td><td>200 J</td></tr><tr><td>Polymorphic VT (irregular form and rate) and unstable</td><td>Treat as VF with high-energy shock (defibrillation doses)</td></tr></table> *Biphasic waveforms using lower energy are acceptable if documented to be clinically equivalent or superior to reports of monophasic shock success. Extrapolation from elective cardioversion of atrial fibrillation supports an initial biphasic dose of 120 J to 200 J with escalation as needed. Consult the device manufacturer for specific recommendations.
8	Announce to team members: "Charging defibrillator—stand clear!"
9	Press the CHARGE button.
10	Clear the patient when the defibrillator is charged. (See "Foundational Facts: Clearing for Defibrillation" in the VF/Pulseless VT Case.)
11	Press the SHOCK button(s).
12	Check the monitor. If tachycardia persists, increase the energy level (joules) according to the Electrical Cardioversion Algorithm.
13	Activate the sync mode after delivery of each synchronized shock. *Most defibrillators default back to the unsynchronized mode after delivery of a synchronized shock. This default allows an immediate shock if cardioversion produces VF.*

Stable Tachycardia Case

Introduction

This case reviews assessment and management of a *stable patient (i.e., no serious signs related to the tachycardia) with a rapid heart rate.* Patients with heart rates >100/min have a tachyarrhythmia or tachycardia. In this case we will use the terms *tachycardia* and *tachyarrhythmia* interchangeably. Note that sinus tachycardia is excluded from the treatment algorithm. Sinus tachycardia is almost always physiologic, developing in response to a compromise in stroke volume or a condition that requires an increase in cardiac output (e.g., fever, hypovolemia). Treatment involves identification and correction of that underlying problem.

You must be able to classify the type of tachycardia (wide or narrow; regular or irregular) and implement appropriate interventions as outlined in the Tachycardia Algorithm. During this case you will:

- Perform initial assessment and management
- Treat regular narrow-complex rhythms (except sinus tachycardia) with vagal maneuvers and adenosine

If the rhythm does not convert, you will monitor the patient and transport or obtain expert consultation. If the patient becomes clinically unstable, you will prepare for immediate unsynchronized shock or synchronized cardioversion as discussed in the Unstable Tachycardia Case.

Learning Objectives

By the end of this case you should be able to:

1. Perform an initial patient assessment to identify symptoms of a stable tachycardia

2. Identify sinus tachycardia

3. State that treatment of sinus tachycardia involves identification of an underlying cause

4. Differentiate between tachycardias with narrow or wide QRS complexes

5. Treat stable tachycardias by using the Tachycardia Algorithm

6. Verbalize when to consider expert consultation

Rhythms for Stable Tachycardia

Tachycardias can be classified in several ways based on the appearance of the QRS |complex, heart rate, and whether they are regular or irregular:

- Narrow–QRS complex (SVT) tachycardias (QRS <0.12 second) in order of frequency
  - Sinus tachycardia
  - Atrial fibrillation
  - Atrial flutter
  - AV nodal reentry
- Wide–QRS complex tachycardias (QRS ≥0.12 second)
  - Monomorphic VT
  - Polymorphic VT
- Regular or irregular tachycardias
  - Irregular narrow-complex tachycardias are probably atrial fibrillation

Drugs for Stable Tachycardia

This case involves the following drug:

- Adenosine

Several agents are also used to provide analgesia and sedation during electrical cardioversion. These agents are not covered in the ACLS Provider Course.

Approach to Stable Tachycardia

Introduction

In this case a stable tachycardia refers to a condition in which the patient has:

- A heart rate >100/min
- No significant signs or symptoms caused by the increased rate
- An underlying cardiac electrical abnormality that generates the rhythm

Questions to Determine Classification

Classification of the tachycardia depends on the careful clinical evaluation of these questions:

- Are symptoms present or absent?
- Are symptoms due to the tachycardia?
- Is the patient stable or unstable?
- Is the QRS complex narrow or wide?
- Is the rhythm regular or irregular?
- Is the QRS monomorphic or polymorphic?
- Is the rhythm sinus tachycardia?

The answers guide subsequent diagnosis and treatment.

Foundational Facts

Understanding Sinus Tachycardia

- Sinus tachycardia is a heart rate that is >100/min and is generated by sinus node discharge. The heart rate in sinus tachycardia does not exceed 220/min and is age-related. Sinus tachycardia usually does not exceed 120 to 130/min, and it has a gradual onset and gradual termination. Reentry SVT has an abrupt onset and termination.

- Sinus tachycardia is caused by *external influences* on the heart, such as fever, anemia, hypotension, blood loss, or exercise. These are systemic conditions, not cardiac conditions. Sinus tachycardia is a regular rhythm, although the rate may be slowed by vagal maneuvers. Cardioversion is contraindicated.

- β-Blockers may cause clinical deterioration if the cardiac output falls when *a compensatory* tachycardia is blocked. This is because cardiac output is determined by the volume of blood ejected by the ventricles with each contraction (stroke volume) and the heart rate.
  Cardiac output (CO) = Stroke volume (SV) × Heart rate

- If a condition such as a large AMI limits ventricular function (severe heart failure or cardiogenic shock), the heart compensates by increasing the heart rate. If you attempt to reduce the heart rate in patients with a compensatory tachycardia, cardiac output will fall and the patient's condition will likely deteriorate.

In sinus tachycardia the goal is to identify and treat the underlying systemic cause.

Managing Stable Tachycardia: The Tachycardia Algorithm

Introduction

As noted in the Unstable Tachycardia Case, the key to management of a patient with any tachycardia is to determine whether pulses are present, and if pulses are present, to determine whether the patient is stable or unstable and then to provide treatment based on patient condition and rhythm. If the patient is pulseless, manage the patient according to the Cardiac Arrest Algorithm (Figure 19, page 61). If the patient has pulses, manage the patient according to the Tachycardia Algorithm (Figure 36, page 127).

Overview

If a tachycardia and a pulse are present, perform assessment and management steps guided by the BLS Survey and the ACLS Survey. Determine if significant symptoms or signs are present and if these symptoms and signs are due to the tachycardia. This will direct you to either the *stable (Boxes 5 through 7)* or *unstable (Box 4)* section of the algorithm.

- If significant signs or symptoms are due to the tachycardia, then the tachycardia is *unstable* and immediate cardioversion is indicated (see the Unstable Tachycardia Case).
- If the patient develops *pulseless VT,* deliver unsynchronized high-energy shocks (defibrillation energy) and follow the Cardiac Arrest Algorithm.
- If the patient has *polymorphic VT,* treat the rhythm as VF and deliver high-energy unsynchronized shocks (i.e., defibrillation energy).

In this case the patient is stable, and you will manage according to the stable section of the Tachycardia Algorithm (Figure 36). A precise identification of the rhythm (e.g., reentry SVT, atrial flutter) may not be possible at this time.

Adult Tachycardia
(With Pulse)

1

Assess appropriateness for clinical condition.
Heart rate typically ≥150/min if tachyarrhythmia.

2

Identify and treat underlying cause

- Maintain patent airway; assist breathing as necessary
- Oxygen (if hypoxemic)
- Cardiac monitor to identify rhythm; monitor blood pressure and oximetry

3

Persistent tachyarrhythmia causing:

- Hypotension?
- Acutely altered mental status?
- Signs of shock?
- Ischemic chest discomfort?
- Acute heart failure?

Yes →

4

Synchronized cardioversion

- Consider sedation
- If regular narrow complex, consider adenosine

No

5

Wide QRS?
≥0.12 second

Yes →

6

- IV access and 12-lead ECG if available
- Consider adenosine only if regular and monomorphic
- Consider antiarrhythmic infusion
- Consider expert consultation

No

7

- IV access and 12-lead ECG if available
- Vagal maneuvers
- Adenosine (if regular)
- β-Blocker or calcium channel blocker
- Consider expert consultation

Doses/Details

Synchronized Cardioversion
Initial recommended doses:
- Narrow regular: 50-100 J
- Narrow irregular: 120-200 J biphasic or 200 J monophasic
- Wide regular: 100 J
- Wide irregular: defibrillation dose (NOT synchronized)

Adenosine IV Dose:
First dose: 6 mg rapid IV push; follow with NS flush.
Second dose: 12 mg if required.

Antiarrhythmic Infusions for Stable Wide-QRS Tachycardia

Procainamide IV Dose:
20-50 mg/min until arrhythmia suppressed, hypotension ensues, QRS duration increases >50%, or maximum dose 17 mg/kg given. Maintenance infusion: 1-4 mg/min. Avoid if prolonged QT or CHF.

Amiodarone IV Dose:
First dose: 150 mg over 10 minutes. Repeat as needed if VT recurs. Follow by maintenance infusion of 1 mg/min for first 6 hours.

Sotalol (not available in Canada) IV Dose:
100 mg (1.5 mg/kg) over 5 minutes. Avoid if prolonged QT.

© 2010 American Heart Association

Figure 36. The Tachycardia With a Pulse Algorithm.

Application of the Tachycardia Algorithm to the Stable Patient

Introduction

In this case a *patient has stable tachycardia with a pulse.* Conduct the steps outlined in the Tachycardia Algorithm to evaluate and manage the patient.

Patient Assessment (Box 1)

Box 1 directs you to assess the patient's condition. Typically, a heart rate >150/min at rest is due to tachyarrhythmias other than sinus tachycardia.

BLS and ACLS Surveys (Box 2)

Using the BLS Survey and the ACLS Survey to guide your approach, evaluate the patient and do the following as necessary:

- Look for signs of increased work of breathing and hypoxia as determined by pulse oximetry.
- Give oxygen; monitor oxygen saturation.
- Support the airway, breathing, and circulation.
- Obtain an ECG to identify the rhythm; check blood pressure.
- Identify and treat reversible causes.

If symptoms persist, proceed to Box 3.

Decision Point: Stable or Unstable (Box 3)

Unstable

If the patient is *unstable* with signs or symptoms as a result of the tachycardia (e.g., hypotension, acutely altered mental status, signs of shock, ischemic chest discomfort, or AHF), go to Box 4 (perform immediate synchronized cardioversion). See the Unstable Tachycardia Case.

Stable

If the patient is stable, go to Box 5.

IV Access and 12-Lead ECG (Box 5)

If the patient with tachycardia is *stable* (i.e., no serious signs or symptoms related to the tachycardia), you have time to evaluate the rhythm and decide on treatment options. Establish IV access if not already obtained. Obtain a 12-lead ECG (when available) or rhythm strip to determine if the QRS is narrow (<0.12 second) or wide (≥0.12 second).

Decision Point: Narrow or Wide (Box 6, Box 7)

The path of treatment is now determined by whether the QRS is wide (Box 6) or narrow (Box 7), and whether the rhythm is regular or irregular. If a monomorphic wide-complex rhythm is present and the patient is stable, expert consultation is advised. Polymorphic wide-complex tachycardia should be treated with immediate unsynchronized cardioversion.

Foundational Facts
Treating Tachycardia

- You may not always be able to distinguish between supraventricular (aberrant) and ventricular wide-complex rhythms. If you are unsure, be aware that most wide-complex (broad-complex) tachycardias are *ventricular* in origin.
- If a patient is *pulseless*, follow the Cardiac Arrest Algorithm.
- If a patient becomes *unstable*, do not delay treatment for further rhythm analysis. For *stable* patients with wide-complex tachycardias, transport and monitor or consult an expert, because treatment has the potential for harm.

Wide (Broad)-Complex Tachycardias (Box 6)

Wide-complex tachycardias are defined as a QRS of ≥0.12 second. *Consider expert consultation.*

The most common forms of life-threatening wide-complex tachycardias likely to deteriorate to VF are:

- Monomorphic VT
- Polymorphic VT

Determine if the rhythm is regular or irregular.

- A regular wide-complex tachycardia is presumed to be VT or SVT with aberrancy.
- An irregular wide-complex tachycardia may be atrial fibrillation with aberrancy, pre-excited atrial fibrillation (atrial fibrillation using an accessory pathway for antegrade conduction), or polymorphic VT/torsades de pointes. These are advanced rhythms requiring additional expertise or expert consultation.

If the rhythm is likely VT or SVT in a stable patient, treat based on the algorithm for that rhythm.

If the rhythm etiology cannot be determined and is regular in its rate and monomorphic, recent evidence suggests that IV adenosine is relatively safe for both treatment and diagnosis. IV antiarrhythmic drugs may be effective. We recommend procainamide, amiodarone, or sotalol. See the right column on the algorithm (Figure 36, page 127) for recommended doses.

In the case of irregular wide-complex tachycardia, management focuses on control of the rapid ventricular rate (rate control), conversion of hemodynamically unstable atrial fibrillation to sinus rhythm (rhythm control), or both. Expert consultation is advised.

Caution **Drugs to Avoid in Patients With Irregular Wide-Complex Tachycardia**	• Avoid AV nodal blocking agents such as adenosine, calcium channel blockers, digoxin, and possibly β-blockers in patients with pre-excitation atrial fibrillation, because these drugs may cause a paradoxical increase in the ventricular response.

Narrow QRS, Regular Rhythm (Box 7)

The therapy for narrow QRS with regular rhythm is:

- Attempt vagal maneuvers
- Give adenosine

Vagal maneuvers and adenosine are the preferred initial interventions for terminating narrow-complex tachycardias that are symptomatic and supraventricular in origin (SVT). Vagal maneuvers alone (Valsalva maneuver or carotid sinus massage) will terminate about 25% of SVTs. Adenosine is required for the remainder.

If SVT does not respond to vagal maneuvers:

- Give **adenosine** 6 mg as a rapid IV push in a large (e.g., antecubital) vein over 1 second. Follow with a 20 mL saline flush and elevate the arm immediately.
- If SVT does not convert within 1 to 2 minutes, give a second dose of adenosine 12 mg rapid IV push following the same procedure above.

Adenosine increases AV block and will terminate approximately 90% of reentry arrhythmias within 2 minutes. Adenosine will not terminate atrial flutter or atrial fibrillation but will slow AV conduction, allowing for identification of flutter or fibrillation waves.

Adenosine is safe and effective in pregnancy. Adenosine does, however, have several important drug interactions. Larger doses may be required for patients with significant blood levels of theophylline, caffeine, or theobromine. The initial dose should be reduced to 3 mg in patients taking dipyridamole or carbamazepine. There have been recent case reports of prolonged asystole following adenosine administration to patients with transplanted hearts or following central venous administration, so lower doses such as 3 mg may be considered in these situations.

Adenosine may cause bronchospasm; therefore, adenosine should not be given to patients with asthma.

If the rhythm converts with adenosine, it is probable reentry SVT. Observe for recurrence. Treat recurrence with adenosine or longer-acting AV nodal blocking agents such as the non-dihydropyridine calcium channel blockers (verapamil and diltiazem) or β-blockers. Typically you should obtain expert consultation if the tachycardia recurs.

If the rhythm does not convert with adenosine, it is possible atrial flutter, ectopic atrial tachycardia, or junctional tachycardia. Obtain expert consultation about diagnosis and treatment.

Caution: **What to Avoid With AV Nodal Blocking Agents**	• AV nodal blocking drugs should not be used for pre-excited atrial fibrillation or flutter. Treatment with an AV nodal blocking agent is unlikely to slow the ventricular rate and in some instances may accelerate the ventricular response. Caution is advised when combining AV nodal blocking agents that have a longer duration of action, such as calcium channel blockers or β-blockers, because their actions may overlap if given serially, which can provoke profound bradycardia.

Tachycardia Algorithm: Advanced Management Steps

Some ACLS providers may be familiar with the differential diagnosis and therapy of stable tachycardias that do not respond to initial treatment. The basic ACLS provider is expected to recognize a stable narrow-complex or wide-complex tachycardia and classify the rhythm as regular or irregular. Regular narrow-complex tachycardias may be treated initially with vagal maneuvers and adenosine. If these are unsuccessful, the ACLS provider should transport or *seek expert consultation*.

If ACLS providers have experience with the differential diagnosis and therapy of stable tachycardias beyond initial management, the Tachycardia Algorithm lists additional steps and pharmacologic agents used in the treatment of these arrhythmias, both for rate control and for termination of the arrhythmia.

> *If at any point you become uncertain or uncomfortable during the treatment of a stable patient, seek expert consultation. The treatment of stable patients may await expert consultation because treatment has the potential for harm.*

Acute Stroke Case

Introduction

The identification and initial management of patients with acute stroke is within the scope of an ACLS provider. This case covers *principles of out-of-hospital care* and *fundamental aspects of initial in-hospital acute stroke care*.

Out-of-hospital acute stroke care focuses on:

- Rapid identification and assessment of patients with stroke
- Rapid transport (with prearrival notification) to a facility capable of providing acute stroke care

In-hospital acute stroke care includes the:

- Ability to rapidly determine patient eligibility for fibrinolytic therapy
- Administration of fibrinolytic therapy to appropriate candidates, with availability of neurologic medical supervision within target times
- Initiation of the stroke pathway and patient admission to a stroke unit if available

The target times and goals are recommended by the National Institute of Neurological Disorders and Stroke (NINDS), which has recommended measurable goals for the evaluation of stroke patients. These targets or goals should be achieved for at least 80% of patients with acute stroke.

Learning Objectives

By the end of this case you should be able to:

1. Describe the major signs and symptoms of stroke

2. Classify strokes to explain stroke type–specific treatments

3. Demonstrate the use of one of the out-of-hospital stroke scales (screening tools) to identify patients with suspected stroke

4. Apply the 8 D's of Stroke Care

5. Explain why timely action is crucial when someone experiences a stroke

6. Follow the Suspected Stroke Algorithm: NINDS time goals

7. Describe why rapid transport to a healthcare facility capable of providing acute stroke care is recommended

8. Recall general eligibility criteria for fibrinolytic therapy

9. Activate the stroke team

Potential Arrhythmias With Stroke

The ECG does not take priority over obtaining a computed tomography (CT) scan. No arrhythmias are specific for stroke, but the ECG may identify evidence of a recent AMI or arrhythmias such as atrial fibrillation as a cause of an embolic stroke. Many patients with stroke may demonstrate arrhythmias, but if the patient is hemodynamically stable, most arrhythmias will not require treatment. There is general agreement to recommend cardiac monitoring during the first 24 hours of evaluation in patients with acute ischemic stroke to detect atrial fibrillation and potentially life-threatening arrhythmias.

Drugs for Stroke

This case involves these drugs:

- Approved fibrinolytic agent (rtPA)
- Glucose (D_{50})
- Labetalol
- Nicardipine
- Enalaprilat
- Aspirin
- Nitroprusside

Foundational Facts
Major Types of Stroke

Stroke is a general term. It refers to acute neurologic impairment that follows interruption in blood supply to a specific area of the brain. Although expeditious stroke care is important for all patients, this case emphasizes reperfusion therapy for acute ischemic stroke.

The major types of stroke are:

- Ischemic stroke: accounts for approximately 80% of all strokes in Canada and is usually caused by an occlusion of an artery to a region of the brain (Figure 37).
- Hemorrhagic stroke: accounts for approximately 20% of all strokes in Canada and occurs when a blood vessel in the brain suddenly ruptures into the surrounding tissue. Fibrinolytic therapy is contraindicated in this type of stroke. Avoid anticoagulants.

Figure 37. Types of stroke. Approximately 80 percent of strokes in Canada are ischemic and potentially eligible for fibrinolytic therapy if patients otherwise qualify. Approximately 20 percent of strokes in Canada are hemorrhagic.

Approach to Stroke Care

Introduction

There are over 50 000 strokes in Canada each year. Stroke remains a leading cause of death in Canada.

Early recognition of acute ischemic stroke is important because IV fibrinolytic treatment should be provided as early as possible, generally within 3 hours of onset of symptoms, or within 4.5 hours of onset of symptoms for selected patients. Most strokes occur at home, and only half of acute stroke patients use EMS for transport to the hospital. Stroke patients often deny or try to rationalize their symptoms. Even high-risk patients, such as those with atrial fibrillation or hypertension, fail to recognize the signs of stroke. This delays activation of EMS and treatment, resulting in increased morbidity and mortality.

Community and professional education is essential, and it has been successful in increasing the proportion of eligible stroke patients treated with fibrinolytic therapy. Healthcare providers, hospitals, and communities must continue to develop systems to improve the efficiency and effectiveness of stroke care.

Foundational Facts
Stroke Chain of Survival

The goal of stroke care is to minimize brain injury and maximize the patient's recovery. The Stroke Chain of Survival (Figure 38) is similar to the Chain of Survival for sudden cardiac arrest. It links actions to be taken by patients, family members, and healthcare providers to maximize stroke recovery. These links are:

- Rapid recognition and reaction to stroke warning signs
- Rapid EMS dispatch
- Rapid EMS system transport and prearrival notification to the receiving hospital
- Rapid diagnosis and treatment in the hospital

Figure 38. The Stroke Chain of Survival.

FYI 2010 Guidelines **Stroke Chain of Survival**	• The background and icons in the figure depicting the stroke Chain of Survival (Figure 38) differ slightly from those in the figure published in the 2006 edition of the *ACLS Provider Manual.* The figure was revised to enhance memorization and avoid confusion with the adult Chain of Survival (Figure 6, page 26), which is new to the 2011 edition of the Provider Manual.

Foundational Facts **The 8 D's of Stroke Care**	The 8 D's of Stroke Care highlight the major steps in diagnosis and treatment of stroke and key points at which delays can occur: • **Detection:** Rapid recognition of stroke symptoms • **Dispatch:** Early activation and dispatch of EMS by 911 • **Delivery:** Rapid EMS identification, management, and transport • **Door:** Appropriate triage to stroke center • **Data:** Rapid triage, evaluation, and management within the ED • **Decision:** Stroke expertise and therapy selection • **Drug:** Fibrinolytic therapy, intra-arterial strategies • **Disposition:** Rapid admission to the stroke unit or critical care unit For more information on these critical elements, see the Suspected Stroke Algorithm (Figure 39).

Goals of Stroke Care

The Suspected Stroke Algorithm (Figure 39) emphasizes important elements of out-of-hospital care for possible stroke patients. These actions include a stroke scale or screen and rapid transport to the hospital. As with ACS, prior notification of the receiving hospital speeds the care of the stroke patient upon arrival.

The NINDS has established critical in-hospital time goals for assessment and management of patients with suspected stroke. This algorithm reviews the critical in-hospital time periods for patient assessment and treatment:

1. Immediate general assessment by the stroke team, emergency physician, or another expert within *10 minutes* of arrival; order urgent noncontrast CT scan

2. Neurologic assessment by the stroke team or designee and CT scan performed within *25 minutes* of hospital arrival

3. Interpretation of the CT scan within *45 minutes* of ED arrival

4. Initiation of fibrinolytic therapy in appropriate patients (those without contraindications) within *1 hour* of hospital arrival and *3 hours* from symptom onset

5. Door-to-admission time of *3 hours*

Adult Suspected Stroke

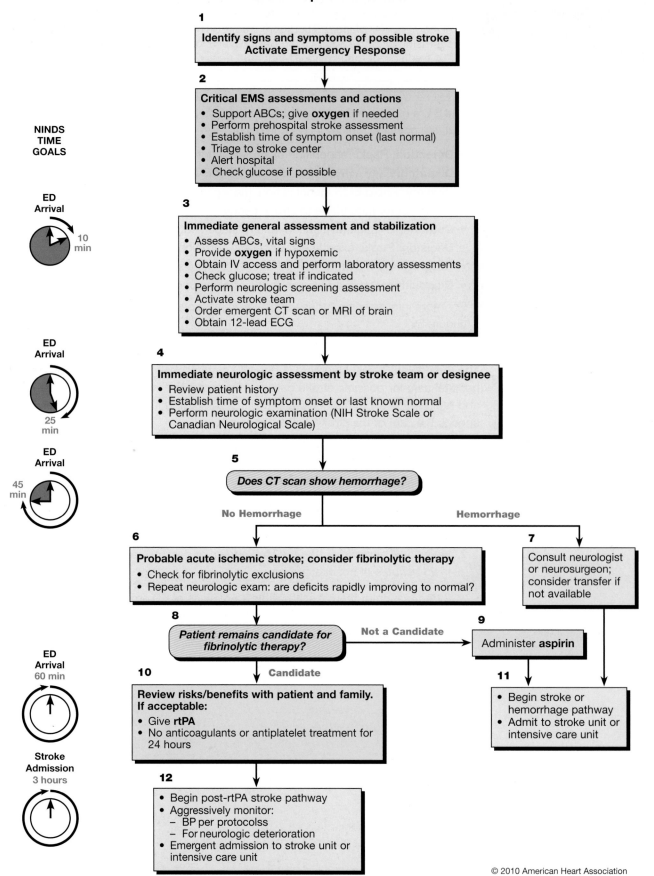

NINDS TIME GOALS

ED Arrival 10 min

ED Arrival 25 min

ED Arrival 45 min

ED Arrival 60 min

Stroke Admission 3 hours

1
Identify signs and symptoms of possible stroke
Activate Emergency Response

2
Critical EMS assessments and actions
• Support ABCs; give **oxygen** if needed
• Perform prehospital stroke assessment
• Establish time of symptom onset (last normal)
• Triage to stroke center
• Alert hospital
• Check glucose if possible

3
Immediate general assessment and stabilization
• Assess ABCs, vital signs
• Provide **oxygen** if hypoxemic
• Obtain IV access and perform laboratory assessments
• Check glucose; treat if indicated
• Perform neurologic screening assessment
• Activate stroke team
• Order emergent CT scan or MRI of brain
• Obtain 12-lead ECG

4
Immediate neurologic assessment by stroke team or designee
• Review patient history
• Establish time of symptom onset or last known normal
• Perform neurologic examination (NIH Stroke Scale or Canadian Neurological Scale)

5
Does CT scan show hemorrhage?

No Hemorrhage   Hemorrhage

6
Probable acute ischemic stroke; consider fibrinolytic therapy
• Check for fibrinolytic exclusions
• Repeat neurologic exam: are deficits rapidly improving to normal?

7
Consult neurologist or neurosurgeon; consider transfer if not available

8
Patient remains candidate for fibrinolytic therapy?   Not a Candidate

9
Administer **aspirin**

Candidate

10
Review risks/benefits with patient and family. If acceptable:
• Give **rtPA**
• No anticoagulants or antiplatelet treatment for 24 hours

11
• Begin stroke or hemorrhage pathway
• Admit to stroke unit or intensive care unit

12
• Begin post-rtPA stroke pathway
• Aggressively monitor:
  – BP per protocolss
  – For neurologic deterioration
• Emergent admission to stroke unit or intensive care unit

© 2010 American Heart Association

Figure 39. The Suspected Stroke Algorithm.

Foundational Facts: The National Institute of Neurological Disorders and Stroke	• The NINDS is a branch of the National Institutes of Health (NIH). Its mission is to reduce the burden of neurologic disease by supporting and conducting research. NINDS researchers have studied stroke and reviewed data leading to recommendations for acute stroke care. The NINDS has set critical time goals for assessment and management of stroke patients based on experience obtained in large studies of stroke patients.

Critical Time Periods

Patients with acute ischemic stroke have a time-dependent benefit for fibrinolytic therapy similar to that of patients with ST-segment elevation MI, but this time-dependent benefit is much shorter.

The critical time period for administration of *IV* fibrinolytic therapy begins with the onset of symptoms. Critical time periods from hospital arrival are summarized below:

Immediate general assessment	10 minutes
Immediate neurologic assessment	25 minutes
Acquisition of CT of the head	25 minutes
Interpretation of the CT scan	45 minutes
Administration of fibrinolytic therapy, timed from ED arrival	60 minutes
Administration of fibrinolytic therapy, timed from onset of symptoms	3 hours, or 4.5 hours in selected patients
Admission to a monitored bed	3 hours

Application of the Suspected Stroke Algorithm

We will now discuss the steps in the algorithm, as well as other related topics:

- Identification of signs and symptoms of possible stroke and activation of emergency response (Box 1)
- Critical EMS assessments and actions (Box 2)
- Immediate general assessment and stabilization (Box 3)
- Immediate neurologic assessment by the stroke team or designee (Box 4)
- CT scan: hemorrhage or no hemorrhage (Box 5)
- Fibrinolytic therapy risk stratification if candidate (Boxes 6, 8, and 10)
- General stroke care (Boxes 11 and 12)

Identification of Signs of Possible Stroke (Box 1)

Warning Signs and Symptoms

The signs and symptoms of a stroke may be subtle. They include:

- Sudden weakness or numbness of the face, arm, or leg, especially on one side of the body
- Sudden confusion
- Trouble speaking or understanding
- Sudden trouble seeing in one or both eyes
- Sudden trouble walking
- Dizziness or loss of balance or coordination
- Sudden severe headache with no known cause

Activate EMS System Immediately

Stroke patients and their families must be educated to activate EMS as soon as they detect potential signs or symptoms of stroke. Currently half of all stroke patients are driven to the ED by family or friends.

EMS provides the safest and most efficient method of emergency transport to the hospital. The advantages of EMS transport include the following:

- EMS personnel can identify and transport a stroke patient to a hospital capable of providing acute stroke care and notify the hospital of the patient's impending arrival.
- Prearrival notification allows the hospital to prepare to evaluate and manage the patient efficiently.

Emergency medical dispatchers also play a critical role in timely treatment of potential stroke by:

- Identifying possible stroke patients
- Providing high-priority dispatch
- Instructing bystanders in lifesaving CPR skills or other supportive care if needed while EMS providers are on the way

Stroke Assessment Tools

The *2010 Guidelines for CPR and ECC* recommends that all EMS personnel be trained to recognize stroke using a validated, abbreviated out-of-hospital neurologic evaluation tool such as the Cincinnati Prehospital Stroke Scale (CPSS) (Table 4).

Cincinnati Prehospital Stroke Scale

The CPSS identifies stroke on the basis of 3 physical findings:

- Facial droop (have the patient smile or try to show teeth)
- Arm drift (have the patient close eyes and hold both arms out, with palms up)
- Abnormal speech (have the patient say "You can't teach an old dog new tricks")

By using the CPSS, medical personnel can evaluate the patient in <1 minute. The presence of 1 finding on the CPSS has a sensitivity of 59% and a specificity of 89% when scored by prehospital providers.

With standard training in stroke recognition, paramedics demonstrated a sensitivity of 61% to 66% for identifying patients with stroke. After receiving training in use of a stroke assessment tool, paramedic sensitivity for identifying patients with stroke increased to 86% to 97%.

Table 4. The Cincinnati Prehospital Stroke Scale

Test	Findings
Facial droop: Have patient show teeth or smile (Figure 40)	• **Normal**—both sides of face move equally • **Abnormal**—one side of face does not move as well as the other side
Arm drift: Patient closes eyes and extends both arms straight out, with palms up, for 10 seconds (Figure 41)	• **Normal**—both arms move the same or both arms do not move at all (other findings, such as pronator drift, may be helpful) • **Abnormal**—one arm does not move or one arm drifts down compared with the other
Abnormal speech: Have patient say "you can't teach an old dog new tricks"	• **Normal**—patient uses correct words with no slurring • **Abnormal**—patient slurs words, uses the wrong words, or is unable to speak
Interpretation: If any 1 of these 3 signs is abnormal, the probability of a stroke is 72%. The presence of all 3 findings indicates that the probability of stroke is >85%.	

Modified from Kothari RU, Pancioli A, Liu T, Brott T, Broderick J. Cincinnati Prehospital Stroke Scale: reproducibility and validity. *Ann Emergency Med.* 1999;33:373-378. With permission from Elsevier.

Figure 40. Facial droop.

Figure 41. One-sided motor weakness (right arm).

Critical EMS Assessments and Actions (Box 2)

Introduction

Prehospital EMS providers must minimize the interval between the onset of symptoms and patient arrival in the ED. Specific stroke therapy can be provided only in the appropriate receiving hospital ED, so time in the field only delays (and may prevent) definitive therapy. More extensive assessments and initiation of supportive therapies can continue en route to the hospital or in the ED.

Critical EMS Assessments and Actions (Box 2)

To provide the best outcome for the patient with potential stroke:

Identify Signs	Define and Recognize the Signs of Stroke (Box 1)
Support ABCs	Support the ABCs and provide supplemental oxygen to hypoxemic (e.g., oxygen saturation <94%) stroke patients or those patients with unknown oxygen saturation.
Perform stroke assessment	Perform a rapid out-of-hospital stroke assessment (CPSS, Table 4).
Establish time	Determine when the patient was last known to be normal or at neurologic baseline. This represents time zero. If the patient wakes from sleep with symptoms of stroke, time zero is the last time the patient was seen to be normal.
Triage to stroke center	Transport the patient rapidly and consider triage to a stroke center. Support cardiopulmonary function during transport. If possible, bring a witness, family member, or caregiver with the patient to confirm time of onset of stroke symptoms.

(continued)

(*continued*)

Identify Signs	Define and Recognize the Signs of Stroke (Box 1)
Alert hospital	Provide prearrival notification to the receiving hospital.
Check glucose	During transport, check blood glucose if protocols or medical control allows.

The patient with acute stroke is at risk for respiratory compromise from aspiration, upper airway obstruction, hypoventilation, and (rarely) neurogenic pulmonary edema. The combination of poor perfusion and hypoxemia will exacerbate and extend ischemic brain injury, and it has been associated with worse outcome from stroke.

Both out-of-hospital and in-hospital medical personnel should provide supplementary oxygen to hypoxemic (i.e., oxygen saturation <94%) stroke patients or patients for whom oxygen saturation is unknown.

Foundational Facts
Stroke Centers and Stroke Units

Initial evidence indicates a favorable benefit from triage of stroke patients directly to designated stroke centers, but the concept of routine out-of-hospital triage of stroke patients requires continued evaluation.

Each receiving hospital should define its capability for treating patients with acute stroke and should communicate this information to the EMS system and the community. Although not every hospital has the resources to safely administer fibrinolytics, every hospital with an ED should have a written plan that describes how patients with acute stroke will be managed in that institution. The plan should:

- Detail the roles of healthcare providers in the care of patients with acute stroke, including identifying sources of neurologic expertise
- Define which patients to treat with fibrinolytics at that facility
- Describe when patient transfer to another hospital with a dedicated stroke unit is appropriate

Patients with stroke who require hospitalization should be admitted to a stroke unit when a stroke unit with a multidisciplinary team experienced in managing stroke is available within a reasonable transport interval.

Studies have documented improvement in 1-year survival rate, functional outcomes, and quality of life when patients hospitalized for acute stroke receive care in a dedicated unit with a specialized team.

In-Hospital, Immediate General Assessment and Stabilization (Box 3)

Introduction

Once the patient arrives in the ED, a number of assessments and management activities must occur quickly. Protocols should be used to minimize delay in definitive diagnosis and therapy.

*The goal of the stroke team, emergency physician, or other experts should be to assess the patient with suspected stroke within **10 minutes of arrival** in the ED: "Time Is Brain" (Box 3).*

Immediate General Assessment and Stabilization

ED providers should do the following:

Step	Actions
Assess ABCs	Assess the ABCs and evaluate baseline vital signs.
Provide oxygen	Provide supplemental oxygen to hypoxemic (e.g., oxyhemoglobin saturation <94%) stroke patients or those patients with unknown oxygen saturation.
Establish IV access and obtain blood samples	Establish IV access and obtain blood samples for baseline blood count, coagulation studies, and blood glucose. Do not let this delay obtaining a CT scan of the brain.
Check glucose	Promptly treat hypoglycemia.
Perform neurologic assessment	Perform a neurologic screening assessment. Use the NIH Stroke Scale (NIHSS) or a similar tool.
Activate the stroke team	Activate the stroke team or arrange consultation with a stroke expert based on predetermined protocols.
Order CT brain scan	Order an emergent CT scan of the brain. Have it read promptly by a qualified physician.
Obtain 12-lead ECG	Obtain a 12-lead ECG, which may identify a recent or ongoing AMI or arrhythmias (e.g., atrial fibrillation) as a cause of embolic stroke. A small percentage of patients with acute stroke or transient ischemic attack have coexisting myocardial ischemia or other abnormalities. There is general agreement to recommend cardiac monitoring during the first 24 hours of evaluation in patients with acute ischemic stroke to detect atrial fibrillation and potentially life-threatening arrhythmias. Life-threatening arrhythmias can follow or accompany stroke, particularly intracerebral hemorrhage. If the patient is hemodynamically stable, treatment of non–life-threatening arrhythmias (bradycardia, VT, and AV conduction blocks) may not be necessary. ***Do not delay the CT scan to obtain the ECG.***

Immediate Neurologic Assessment by Stroke Team or Designee (Box 4)

Overview

The stroke team, neurovascular consultant, or emergency physician does the following:

- Reviews the patient's history, performs a general physical examination, and establishes time of symptom onset
- Performs a neurologic examination (e.g., NIHSS)

The goal for neurologic assessment is within 25 minutes of the patient's arrival in the ED: "Time Is Brain" (Box 4).

Establish Symptom Onset	Establishing the time of symptom onset may require interviewing out-of-hospital providers, witnesses, and family members to determine the time the patient was last known to be normal.

Neurologic Examination	Assess the patient's neurologic status using one of the more advanced stroke scales. Following is an example: **National Institutes of Health Stroke Scale** The NIHSS uses 15 items to assess the responsive stroke patient. This is a validated measure of stroke severity based on a detailed neurologic examination. A detailed discussion is beyond the scope of the ACLS Provider Course.

CT Scan: Hemorrhage or No Hemorrhage (Box 5)

Introduction	A critical decision point in the assessment of the patient with acute stroke is the performance and interpretation of a noncontrast CT scan to differentiate ischemic from hemorrhagic stroke. Assessment also includes identifying other structural abnormalities that may be responsible for the patient's symptoms or that represent contraindication to fibrinolytic therapy. The initial noncontrast CT scan is the most important test for a patient with acute stroke. • If a CT scan is not readily available, stabilize and promptly transfer the patient to a facility with this capability. • Do not give aspirin, heparin, or rtPA until the CT scan has ruled out intracranial hemorrhage. *The CT scan should be completed within 25 minutes of the patient's arrival in the ED and should be read within 45 minutes from ED arrival: "Time Is Brain" (Box 5).*

Decision Point: Hemorrhage or No Hemorrhage	Additional imaging techniques such as CT perfusion, CT angiography, or magnetic resonance imaging scans of patients with suspected stroke should be promptly interpreted by a physician skilled in neuroimaging interpretation. Obtaining these studies should not delay initiation of IV rtPA in eligible patients. The presence of hemorrhage versus no hemorrhage determines the next steps in treatment (Figures 42A and B). ### *Yes, Hemorrhage Is Present* If hemorrhage is noted on the CT scan, the patient is not a candidate for fibrinolytics. Consult a neurologist or neurosurgeon. Consider transfer for appropriate care (Box 7). ### *No, Hemorrhage Is Not Present* If the CT scan shows no evidence of hemorrhage and no sign of other abnormality (e.g., tumor, recent stroke), the patient may be a candidate for fibrinolytic therapy (Boxes 6 and 8). If hemorrhage is not present on the initial CT scan and the patient is not a candidate for fibrinolytics for other reasons, consider giving aspirin (Box 9) either rectally or orally after performing a swallowing screen (see below). Although aspirin is not a time-critical intervention, it is appropriate to administer aspirin in the ED if the patient is not a candidate for fibrinolysis. The patient must be able to safely swallow before aspirin is given orally. Otherwise use the suppository form.

Ischemic Penumbra

Infarcted Brain Tissue

A

B

Figure 42. Occlusion in a cerebral artery by a thrombus. **A.** Area of infarction surrounding immediate site and distal portion of brain tissue after occlusion. **B.** Area of ischemic penumbra (ischemic, but not yet infarcted [dead] brain tissue) surrounding areas of infarction. This ischemic penumbra is alive but dysfunctional because of altered membrane potentials. The dysfunction is potentially reversible. Current stroke treatment tries to keep the area of permanent brain infarction as small as possible by preventing the areas of reversible brain ischemia in the penumbra from transforming into larger areas of irreversible brain infarction.

Fibrinolytic Therapy

Introduction

Several studies have shown a higher likelihood of good to excellent functional outcome when rtPA is given to adults with acute ischemic stroke within 3 hours of onset of symptoms, or within 4.5 hours of onset of symptoms for selected patients. But these results are obtained when rtPA is given by physicians in hospitals with a stroke protocol that rigorously adheres to the eligibility criteria and therapeutic regimen of the NINDS protocol. Evidence from prospective randomized studies in adults also documents a greater likelihood of benefit the earlier treatment begins.

The HSFC and stroke guidelines recommend giving IV rtPA to patients with acute ischemic stroke who meet the NINDS eligibility criteria if it is given by

- Physicians using a clearly defined institutional protocol
- A knowledgeable interdisciplinary team familiar with stroke care
- An institution with a commitment to comprehensive stroke care and rehabilitation

The superior outcomes reported in both community and tertiary care hospitals in the NINDS trials can be difficult to replicate in hospitals with less experience in, and institutional commitment to, acute stroke care. There is strong evidence to avoid all delays and treat patients as soon as possible. Failure to adhere to protocol is associated with an increased rate of complications, particularly risk of intracranial hemorrhage.

Evaluate for Fibrinolytic Therapy (Box 6)

If the CT scan is negative for hemorrhage, the patient may be a candidate for fibrinolytic therapy. Immediately perform further eligibility and risk stratification:

- If the CT scan shows no hemorrhage, the probability of acute ischemic stroke remains. *Review inclusion and exclusion criteria for IV fibrinolytic therapy (Table 5) and repeat the neurologic exam* (NIHSS or Canadian Neurological Scale).
- If the patient's neurologic function is rapidly improving toward normal, fibrinolytics may be unnecessary.

Table 5. Inclusion and Exclusion Characteristics of Patients With Ischemic Stroke Who Could Be Treated With rtPA Within *3 Hours* From Symptom Onset*

Inclusion Criteria
• Diagnosis of ischemic stroke causing measurable neurologic deficit • Onset of symptoms <3 hours before beginning treatment • Age ≥18 years
Exclusion Criteria

• Head trauma or prior stroke in previous 3 months
• Symptoms suggest subarachnoid hemorrhage
• Arterial puncture at noncompressible site in previous 7 days
• History of previous intracranial hemorrhage
• Elevated blood pressure (systolic >185 mm Hg or diastolic >110 mm Hg)
• Evidence of active bleeding on examination
• Acute bleeding diathesis, including but not limited to
   – Platelet count <100 000/mm^3
   – Heparin received within 48 hours, resulting in an aPTT greater than the upper limit of normal
   – Current use of anticoagulant with INR >1.7 or PT >15 seconds
• Blood glucose concentration <50 mg/dL (2.7 mmol/L)
• CT demonstrates multilobar infarction (hypodensity >⅓ cerebral hemisphere)

(continued)

(continued)

Relative Exclusion Criteria
Recent experience suggests that under some circumstances—with careful consideration and weighing of risk to benefit—patients may receive fibrinolytic therapy despite 1 or more relative contraindications. Consider risk to benefit of rtPA administration carefully if any one of these relative contraindications is present:

- Only minor or rapidly improving stroke symptoms (clearing spontaneously)
- Seizure at onset with postictal residual neurologic impairments
- Major surgery or serious trauma within previous 14 days
- Recent gastrointestinal or urinary tract hemorrhage (within previous 21 days)
- Recent acute myocardial infarction (within previous 3 months)

Abbreviations: aPTT, activated partial thromboplastin time; INR, international normalized ratio; PT, prothrombin time; rtPA, recombinant tissue plasminogen activator.

*Adams HP Jr, del Zoppo G, Alberts MJ, Bhatt DL, Brass L, Furlan A, Grubb RL, Higashida RT, Jauch EC, Kidwell C, Lyden PD, Morgenstern LB, Qureshi AI, Rosenwasser RH, Scott PA, Wijdicks EFM. Guidelines for the early management of adults with ischemic stroke: a guideline from the American Heart Association/American Stroke Association Stroke Council, Clinical Cardiology Council, Cardiovascular Radiology and Intervention Council, and the Atherosclerotic Peripheral Vascular Disease and Quality of Care Outcomes in Research Interdisciplinary Working Groups. *Stroke.* 2007;38:1655-1711.

Potential Adverse Effects

As with all drugs, fibrinolytics have potential adverse effects. At this point weigh the patient's risk for adverse events against the potential benefit and discuss with the patient and family.

- Confirm that no exclusion criteria are present (Table 5).
- Consider risks and benefits.
- Be prepared to monitor and treat any potential complications.

The major complication of IV rtPA for stroke is intracranial hemorrhage. Other bleeding complications may occur and may range from minor to major. Angioedema and transient hypotension may occur.

Patient Is a Candidate for Fibrinolytic Therapy (Boxes 8 and 10)

If the patient remains a candidate for fibrinolytic therapy (Box 8), discuss the risks and potential benefits with the patient or family if available (Box 10). After this discussion, if the patient or family members decide to proceed with fibrinolytic therapy, give the patient rtPA. Begin your institution's stroke rtPA protocol, often called a "pathway of care."

> *Do not administer anticoagulants or antiplatelet treatment for 24 hours after administration of rtPA, typically until a follow-up CT scan at 24 hours shows no intracranial hemorrhage.*

Extended IV rtPA Window 3 to 4.5 Hours

Treatment of carefully selected patients with acute ischemic stroke with IV rtPA between 3 and 4.5 hours after onset of symptoms has also been shown to improve clinical outcome, although the degree of clinical benefit is smaller than that achieved with treatment within 3 hours. Data supporting treatment in this time window come from a large, randomized trial (ECASS-3 [European Cooperative Acute Stroke Study]) that specifically enrolled patients between 3 and 4.5 hours after symptom onset, as well as a meta-analysis of prior trials.

Health Canada has approved the clot-busting drug called tPA to be used within 3 hours from the time symptoms begin. However, emerging science is now showing that tPA could be effective up to 4 1/2 hours afterward. As a result, the Canadian Stroke Strategy has issued new Canadian Best Practices Recommendations for Stroke Care, which have included this new treatment time. Still, it will be up to the attending emergency doctors to determine when tPA may be administered or if it is appropriate to the situation. Administration of IV rtPA to patients with acute ischemic stroke who meet the NINDS or ECASS-3 eligibility criteria (Table 6) is recommended if rtPA is administered by physicians in the setting of a clearly defined protocol, a knowledgeable team, and institutional commitment.

Table 6. Inclusion and Exclusion Characteristics of Patients With Ischemic Stroke Who Could Be Treated With rtPA From 3 to 4.5 Hours From Symptom Onset*

Inclusion Criteria
• Diagnosis of ischemic stroke causing measurable neurologic deficit • Onset of symptoms 3 to 4.5 hours before beginning treatment
Exclusion Criteria
• Age >80 years • Severe stroke (NIHSS >25) • Taking an oral anticoagulant regardless of INR • History of both diabetes and prior ischemic stroke
Notes • A physician with expertise in acute stroke care may modify this list. • Onset time is either witnessed or last known normal. • In patients without recent use of oral anticoagulants or heparin, treatment with rtPA can be initiated before availability of coagulation study results but should be discontinued if INR is >1.7 or PT is elevated by local laboratory standards. • In patients without a history of thrombocytopenia, treatment with rtPA can be initiated before availability of platelet count but should be discontinued if platelet count is <100 000/mm³.

Abbreviations: FDA, Food and Drug Administration; INR, international normalized ratio; NIHSS, National Institutes of Health Stroke Scale; PT, prothrombin time; rtPA, recombinant tissue plasminogen activator.

*del Zoppo GJ, Saver JL, Jauch EC, Adams HP Jr; on behalf of the American Heart Association Stroke Council. Expansion of the time window for treatment of acute ischemic stroke with intravenous tissue plasminogen activator: a science advisory from the American Heart Association/American Stroke Association. *Stroke.* 2009;40:2945-2948.

Intra-arterial rtPA

Improved outcome from use of cerebral intra-arterial rtPA has been documented. For patients with acute ischemic stroke who are not candidates for standard IV fibrinolysis, consider intra-arterial fibrinolysis in centers with the resources and expertise to provide it within the first 6 hours after onset of symptoms. Intra-arterial administration of rtPA is not yet approved by the FDA.

General Stroke Care (Boxes 11 and 12)

Introduction

The general care of all patients with stroke includes the following:

- Begin stroke pathway.
- Support airway, breathing, and circulation.
- Monitor blood glucose.
- Monitor blood pressure.
- Monitor temperature.
- Perform dysphagia screening.
- Monitor for complications of stroke and fibrinolytic therapy.
- Transfer to general intensive care if indicated.

Begin Stroke Pathway (Boxes 11 and 12)

Admit patients to a stroke unit (if available) for careful observation (Box 11), including monitoring of blood pressure and neurologic status. If neurologic status worsens, order an emergent CT scan. Determine if cerebral edema or hemorrhage is the cause; consult neurosurgery as appropriate.

Additional stroke care includes support of the airway, oxygenation, ventilation, and nutrition. Provide normal saline to maintain intravascular volume (e.g., approximately 75 to 100 mL/h) if needed.

Monitor Blood Glucose

Hyperglycemia is associated with worse clinical outcome in patients with acute ischemic stroke. But there is no direct evidence that active glucose control improves clinical outcome. There is evidence that insulin treatment of hyperglycemia in other critically ill patients improves survival rates. For this reason, consider giving IV or subcutaneous insulin to lower blood glucose in patients with acute ischemic stroke when the serum glucose level is >185 mg/dL (10 mmol/L).

Monitor for Complications of Stroke and Fibrinolytic Therapy

Prophylaxis for seizures is not recommended. But treatment of acute seizures followed by administration of anticonvulsants to prevent further seizures is recommended. Monitor the patient for signs of increased intracranial pressure. Continue to control blood pressure to reduce the potential risk of bleeding.

Hypertension Management in rtPA Candidates

Although management of hypertension in the stroke patient is controversial, patients who are candidates for fibrinolytic therapy should have their blood pressure controlled to lower the risk of intracerebral hemorrhage following administration of rtPA. General guidelines for the management of hypertension are outlined in Tables 7 and 8.

If patient is eligible for fibrinolytic therapy, blood pressure must be ≤185 mm Hg systolic and ≤110 mm Hg diastolic to limit the risk of bleeding complications. Because the maximum interval from onset of stroke until effective treatment of stroke with rtPA is limited, most patients with sustained hypertension above these levels will not be eligible for IV rtPA.

Table 7. Potential Approaches to Arterial Hypertension in Patients With Acute Ischemic Stroke Who Are Potential Candidates for Acute Reperfusion Therapy*

Patient otherwise eligible for acute reperfusion therapy except that blood pressure is >185/110 mm Hg:

- Labetalol 10-20 mg IV over 1-2 minutes, may repeat × 1, or
- Nicardipine IV 5 mg per hour, titrate up by 2.5 mg per hour every 5-15 minutes, maximum 15 mg per hour; when desired blood pressure is reached, lower to 3 mg per hour, or
- Other agents (hydralazine, enalaprilat, etc) may be considered when appropriate

If blood pressure is not maintained at or below 185/110 mm Hg, do not administer rtPA.

Management of blood pressure during and after rtPA or other acute reperfusion therapy:

Monitor blood pressure every 15 minutes for 2 hours from the start of rtPA therapy, then every 30 minutes for 6 hours, and then every hour for 16 hours.

If systolic blood pressure 180-230 mm Hg or diastolic blood pressure 105-120 mm Hg:

- Labetalol 10 mg IV followed by continuous IV infusion 2-8 mg per minute, or
- Nicardipine IV 5 mg per hour, titrate up to desired effect by 2.5 mg per hour every 5-15 minutes, maximum 15 mg per hour

If blood pressure not controlled or diastolic blood pressure >140 mm Hg, consider sodium nitroprusside.

*Adams HP Jr, del Zoppo G, Alberts MJ, Bhatt DL, Brass L, Furlan A, Grubb RL, Higashida RT, Jauch EC, Kidwell C, Lyden PD, Morgenstern LB, Qureshi AI, Rosenwasser RH, Scott PA, Wijdicks EFM. Guidelines for the early management of adults with ischemic stroke: a guideline from the American Heart Association/ American Stroke Association Stroke Council, Clinical Cardiology Council, Cardiovascular Radiology and Intervention Council, and the Atherosclerotic Peripheral Vascular Disease and Quality of Care Outcomes in Research Interdisciplinary Working Groups. *Stroke.* 2007;38:1655-1711.

Table 8. Approach to Arterial Hypertension in Patients With Acute Ischemic Stroke Who Are *Not* Potential Candidates for Acute Reperfusion Therapy*

Consider lowering blood pressure in patients with acute ischemic stroke if systolic blood pressure >220 mm Hg or diastolic blood pressure >120 mm Hg.

Consider blood pressure reduction as indicated for other concomitant organ system injury:

- Acute myocardial infarction
- Congestive heart failure
- Acute aortic dissection

A reasonable target is to lower blood pressure by 15% to 25% within the first day.

*Adams HP Jr, del Zoppo G, Alberts MJ, Bhatt DL, Brass L, Furlan A, Grubb RL, Higashida RT, Jauch EC, Kidwell C, Lyden PD, Morgenstern LB, Qureshi AI, Rosenwasser RH, Scott PA, Wijdicks EFM. Guidelines for the early management of adults with ischemic stroke: a guideline from the American Heart Association/ American Stroke Association Stroke Council, Clinical Cardiology Council, Cardiovascular Radiology and Intervention Council, and the Atherosclerotic Peripheral Vascular Disease and Quality of Care Outcomes in Research Interdisciplinary Working Groups. *Stroke.* 2007;38:1655-1711.

Appendix

Management of Respiratory Arrest
Bag-Mask Ventilation Testing Checklist

Student Name: _____ Test Date: _____

Performance Guidelines and Critical Actions	✓ if done correctly
BLS Survey and Interventions	
Checks for responsiveness • Taps and shouts, "Are you all right?" *and* • Scans chest for movement (5-10 seconds)	
Activates the emergency response system • Activates the emergency response system and gets the AED *or* • Directs second rescuer to activate the emergency response system and get the AED	
Checks carotid pulse (5-10 seconds). Notes that pulse is present Does not initiate chest compressions or attach AED Performs ventilations at the correct rate of 1 breath every 5-6 seconds (10-12 breaths per minute)	
ACLS Survey Case Skills	
Inserts oropharyngeal or nasopharyngeal airway	
Administers oxygen	
Performs correct bag-mask ventilation for 1 minute	
Critical Actions	
Effectively ventilates with a bag-mask device for 1 minute	
Gives proper ventilation—rate and volume	

STOP TEST

Test Results	Circle P or NR to Indicate Pass or Needs Remediation:	P	NR
Instructor signature affirms that skills tests were done according to HSFC Guidelines. *Save this sheet with course record.*	Instructor Signature: _____ Print Instructor Name: _____ Date: _____		

CPR and AED Skills Test
1-Rescuer Adult CPR and AED Checklist

Student Name: _____ Test Date: _____

Skill Step	Critical Performance Steps	✓ if done correctly
BLS Survey and Interventions		
1	Checks for responsiveness: *Taps and shouts, "Are you all right?" and scans the chest for movement (5-10 seconds)*	
2	Tells someone to activate the emergency response system and get an AED	
3	Checks carotid pulse *(minimum 5 seconds; maximum 10 seconds)*	
4	Bares patient's chest and locates CPR hand position	
5	Delivers first cycle of compressions at correct rate *(acceptable: 18 seconds or less for 30 compressions)*	
6	Gives 2 breaths (1 second each)	
AED Arrives		
AED 1	Turns AED on, selects proper pads, and places pads correctly	
AED 2	Clears patient to analyze *(must be visible and verbal check)*	
AED 3	Clears patient to shock/presses shock button *(must be visible and verbal check; maximum time from AED arrival less than 45 seconds)*	
Student Continues CPR		
7	Delivers second cycle of compressions at correct hand position *(acceptable: greater than 23 of 30 compressions)*	
8	Gives 2 breaths (1 second each) with visible chest rise	
The next step is performed only if the manikin is equipped with a feedback device, such as a clicker or light. If there is no feedback device, STOP THE TEST.		
9	Delivers third cycle of compressions of adequate depth with complete chest recoil *(acceptable: greater than 23 compressions)*	

STOP TEST

Test Results	Circle P or NR to Indicate Pass or Needs Remediation:	P	NR
Instructor signature affirms that skills tests were done according to HSFC Guidelines. *Save this sheet with course record.*	Instructor Signature: _____ Print Instructor Name: _____ Date: _____		

Megacode Testing Checklist 1/2
Bradycardia → VF/Pulseless VT → Asystole → ROSC

HEART&™
STROKE
FOUNDATION
OF CANADA

Student Name: _____   Test Date: _____

Critical Performance Steps	✓ if done correctly
Team Leader	
Ensures high-quality CPR at all times	
Assigns team member roles	
Ensures that team members perform well	
Bradycardia Management	
Starts oxygen if needed, places monitor, starts IV	
Places monitor leads in proper position	
Recognizes symptomatic bradycardia	
Administers correct dose of atropine	
Prepares for second-line treatment	
VF/Pulseless VT Management	
Recognizes VF	
Clears before ANALYZE and SHOCK	
Immediately resumes CPR after shocks	
Appropriate airway management	
Appropriate cycles of drug–rhythm check/shock–CPR	
Administers appropriate drug(s) and doses	
Asystole Management	
Recognizes asystole	
Verbalizes potential reversible causes of asystole/PEA (H's and T's)	
Administers appropriate drug(s) and doses	
Immediately resumes CPR after rhythm checks	
Post–Cardiac Arrest Care	
Identifies ROSC	
Ensures BP and 12-lead ECG are performed, O_2 saturation is monitored, verbalizes need for endotracheal intubation and waveform capnography, and orders laboratory tests	
Considers therapeutic hypothermia	

STOP TEST

Test Results	Circle P or NR to Indicate Pass or Needs Remediation:	P	NR
Instructor signature affirms that skills tests were done according to HSFC Guidelines. *Save this sheet with course record.*	Instructor Signature: _____ Print Instructor Name: _____ Date: _____		

153

Megacode Testing Checklist 3
Tachycardia → VF/Pulseless VT → PEA → ROSC

Student Name: _____ Test Date: _____

Critical Performance Steps	✓ if done correctly
Team Leader	
Ensures high-quality CPR at all times	
Assigns team member roles	
Ensures that team members perform well	
Tachycardia Management	
Starts oxygen if needed, places monitor, starts IV	
Places monitor leads in proper position	
Recognizes unstable tachycardia	
Recognizes symptoms due to tachycardia	
Performs immediate synchronized cardioversion	
VF/Pulseless VT Management	
Recognizes VF	
Clears before ANALYZE and SHOCK	
Immediately resumes CPR after shocks	
Appropriate airway management	
Appropriate cycles of drug–rhythm check/shock–CPR	
Administers appropriate drug(s) and doses	
PEA Management	
Recognizes PEA	
Verbalizes potential reversible causes of PEA/asystole (H's and T's)	
Administers appropriate drug(s) and doses	
Immediately resumes CPR after rhythm and pulse checks	
Post–Cardiac Arrest Care	
Identifies ROSC	
Ensures BP and 12-lead ECG are performed, O₂ saturation is monitored, verbalizes need for endotracheal intubation and waveform capnography, and orders laboratory tests	
Considers therapeutic hypothermia	

STOP TEST

Test Results	Circle P or NR to Indicate Pass or Needs Remediation:	P	NR
Instructor signature affirms that skills tests were done according to HSFC Guidelines. *Save this sheet with course record.*	Instructor Signature: _____ Print Instructor Name: _____ Date: _____		

Megacode Testing Checklist 4
Tachycardia → VF/Pulseless VT → PEA → ROSC

Student Name: _____ Test Date: _____

Critical Performance Steps	✓ if done correctly
Team Leader	
Ensures high-quality CPR at all times	
Assigns team member roles	
Ensures that team members perform well	
Tachycardia Management	
Starts oxygen if needed, places monitor, starts IV	
Places monitor leads in proper position	
Recognizes tachycardia (specific diagnosis)	
Recognizes no symptoms due to tachycardia	
Attempts vagal maneuvers	
Gives appropriate initial drug therapy	
VF/Pulseless VT Management	
Recognizes VF	
Clears before ANALYZE and SHOCK	
Immediately resumes CPR after shocks	
Appropriate airway management	
Appropriate cycles of drug–rhythm check/shock–CPR	
Administers appropriate drug(s) and doses	
PEA Management	
Recognizes PEA	
Verbalizes potential reversible causes of PEA/asystole (H's and T's)	
Administers appropriate drug(s) and doses	
Immediately resumes CPR after rhythm and pulse checks	
Post–Cardiac Arrest Care	
Identifies ROSC	
Ensures BP and 12-lead ECG are performed, O_2 saturation is monitored, verbalizes need for endotracheal intubation and waveform capnography, and orders laboratory tests	
Considers therapeutic hypothermia	

STOP TEST

Test Results	Circle P or NR to Indicate Pass or Needs Remediation:	P	NR

Instructor signature affirms that skills tests were done according to HSFC Guidelines.

Save this sheet with course record.

Instructor Signature: _____

Print Instructor Name: _____

Date: _____

Megacode Testing Checklist 5
Tachycardia → VF/Pulseless VT → PEA → ROSC

Student Name: _____ Test Date: _____

Critical Performance Steps	✓ if done correctly
Team Leader	
Ensures high-quality CPR at all times	
Assigns team member roles	
Ensures that team members perform well	
Tachycardia Management	
Starts oxygen if needed, places monitor, starts IV	
Places monitor leads in proper position	
Recognizes unstable tachycardia	
Recognizes symptoms due to tachycardia	
Performs immediate synchronized cardioversion	
VF/Pulseless VT Management	
Recognizes VF	
Clears before ANALYZE and SHOCK	
Immediately resumes CPR after shocks	
Appropriate airway management	
Appropriate cycles of drug–rhythm check/shock–CPR	
Administers appropriate drug(s) and doses	
PEA Management	
Recognizes PEA	
Verbalizes potential reversible causes of PEA/asystole (H's and T's)	
Administers appropriate drug(s) and doses	
Immediately resumes CPR after rhythm and pulse checks	
Post–Cardiac Arrest Care	
Identifies ROSC	
Ensures BP and 12-lead ECG are performed, O$_2$ saturation is monitored, verbalizes need for endotracheal intubation and waveform capnography, and orders laboratory tests	
Considers therapeutic hypothermia	

STOP TEST

Test Results	Circle P or NR to Indicate Pass or Needs Remediation:	P	NR
Instructor signature affirms that skills tests were done according to HSFC Guidelines. *Save this sheet with course record.*	Instructor Signature: _____ Print Instructor Name: _____ Date: _____		

Megacode Testing Checklist 6
Tachycardia → VF/Pulseless VT → PEA → ROSC

Student Name: _____ Test Date: _____

Critical Performance Steps	✓ if done correctly
Team Leader	
Ensures high-quality CPR at all times	
Assigns team member roles	
Ensures that team members perform well	
Tachycardia Management	
Starts oxygen if needed, places monitor, starts IV	
Places monitor leads in proper position	
Recognizes tachycardia (specific diagnosis)	
Recognizes no symptoms due to tachycardia	
Attempts vagal maneuvers	
Gives appropriate initial drug therapy	
VF/Pulseless VT Management	
Recognizes VF	
Clears before ANALYZE and SHOCK	
Immediately resumes CPR after shocks	
Appropriate airway management	
Appropriate cycles of drug–rhythm check/shock–CPR	
Administers appropriate drug(s) and doses	
PEA Management	
Recognizes PEA	
Verbalizes potential reversible causes of PEA/asystole (H's and T's)	
Administers appropriate drug(s) and doses	
Immediately resumes CPR after rhythm and pulse checks	
Post–Cardiac Arrest Care	
Identifies ROSC	
Ensures BP and 12-lead ECG are performed, O$_2$ saturation is monitored, verbalizes need for endotracheal intubation and waveform capnography, and orders laboratory tests	
Considers therapeutic hypothermia	

STOP TEST

Test Results	Circle P or NR to Indicate Pass or Needs Remediation:	P	NR
Instructor signature affirms that skills tests were done according to HSFC Guidelines. *Save this sheet with course record.*	Instructor Signature: _____ Print Instructor Name: _____ Date: _____		

Cardiac Arrest VF/Pulseless VT Learning Station Checklist

Adult Cardiac Arrest

☐ Shout for Help/Activate Emergency Response

1 ☐ **Start CPR**
- Give oxygen
- Attach monitor/defibrillator

Rhythm shockable?

Yes ☐

No

2 ☐ **VF/VT**

9 **Asystole/PEA**

3 ⚡ Shock ☐

4 ☐ **CPR 2 min**
- IV/IO access

☐ **Rhythm shockable?** No

Yes

5 ⚡ Shock ☐

6 ☐ **CPR 2 min**
- **Epinephrine** every 3-5 min
- Consider advanced airway, capnography

☐ **Rhythm shockable?** No

Yes

7 ⚡ Shock ☐

8 ☐ **CPR 2 min**
- **Amiodarone**
- Treat reversible causes

10 **CPR 2 min**
- IV/IO access
- **Epinephrine** every 3-5 min
- Consider advanced airway, capnography

Rhythm shockable? Yes

No

11 **CPR 2 min**
- Treat reversible causes

Rhythm shockable? Yes ⟶ **Go to 5 or 7**

No

12 ☐
- If no signs of return of spontaneous circulation (ROSC), go to **10** or **11**
- If ROSC, go to Post–Cardiac Arrest Care

CPR Quality ☐
- Push hard (≥5 cm [2 inches]) and fast (≥100/min) and allow complete chest recoil
- Minimize interruptions in compressions
- Avoid excessive ventilation
- Rotate compressor every 2 minutes
- If no advanced airway, 30:2 compression-ventilation ratio
- Quantitative waveform capnography
  - If P_{ETCO_2} <10 mm Hg, attempt to improve CPR quality
- Intra-arterial pressure
  - If relaxation phase (diastolic) pressure <20 mm Hg, attempt to improve CPR quality

Return of Spontaneous Circulation (ROSC)
- Pulse and blood pressure
- Abrupt sustained increase in P_{ETCO_2} (typically ≥40 mm Hg)
- Spontaneous arterial pressure waves with intra-arterial monitoring

Shock Energy
- **Biphasic:** Manufacturer recommendation (e.g., initial dose of 120-200 J); if unknown, use maximum available. Second and subsequent doses should be equivalent, and higher doses may be considered.
- **Monophasic:** 360 J

Drug Therapy
- **Epinephrine IV/IO Dose:** 1 mg every 3-5 minutes
- **Vasopressin IV/IO Dose:** 40 units can replace first or second dose of epinephrine
- **Amiodarone IV/IO Dose:** First dose: 300 mg bolus. Second dose: 150 mg.

Advanced Airway
- Supraglottic advanced airway or endotracheal intubation
- Waveform capnography to confirm and monitor ET tube placement
- 8-10 breaths per minute with continuous chest compressions

Reversible Causes ☐
- **H**ypovolemia
- **H**ypoxia
- **H**ydrogen ion (acidosis)
- **H**ypo-/hyperkalemia
- **H**ypothermia
- **T**ension pneumothorax
- **T**amponade, cardiac
- **T**oxins
- **T**hrombosis, pulmonary
- **T**hrombosis, coronary

Cardiac Arrest PEA/Asystole Learning Station Checklist

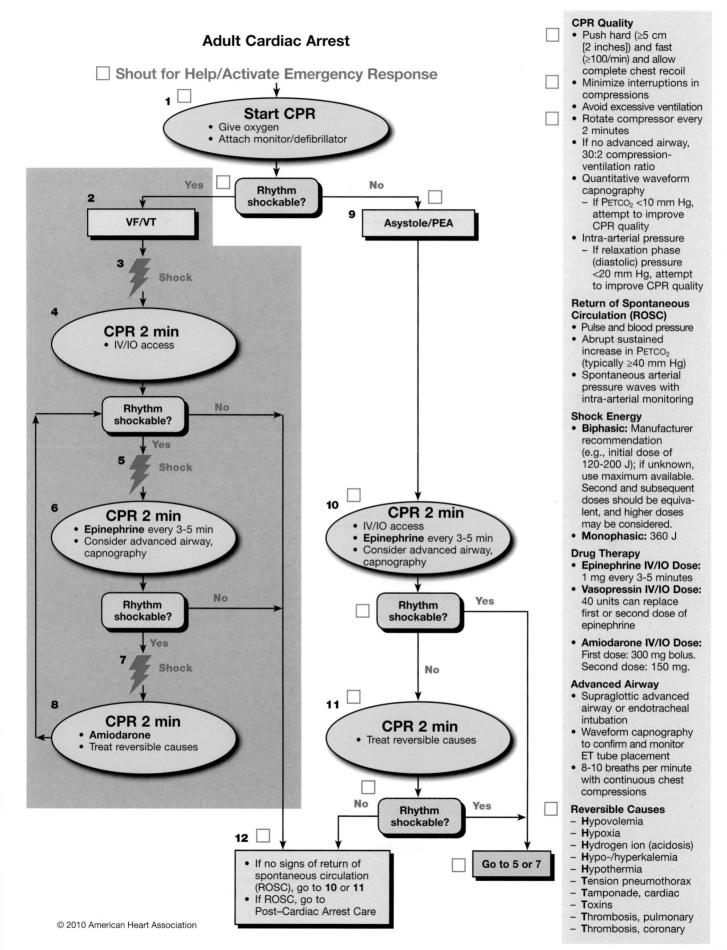

Adult Cardiac Arrest

☐ **Shout for Help/Activate Emergency Response**

1 ☐
Start CPR
- Give oxygen
- Attach monitor/defibrillator

Rhythm shockable? ☐
Yes ☐ / No

2 **VF/VT**

9 **Asystole/PEA** ☐

3 ⚡ Shock

4
CPR 2 min
- IV/IO access

Rhythm shockable? No

Yes

5 ⚡ Shock

6
CPR 2 min
- **Epinephrine** every 3-5 min
- Consider advanced airway, capnography

Rhythm shockable? No

Yes

7 ⚡ Shock

8
CPR 2 min
- **Amiodarone**
- Treat reversible causes

10 ☐
CPR 2 min
- IV/IO access
- **Epinephrine** every 3-5 min
- Consider advanced airway, capnography

Rhythm shockable? ☐ Yes

No

11 ☐
CPR 2 min
- Treat reversible causes

Rhythm shockable? ☐ No / Yes

Go to 5 or 7 ☐

12 ☐
- If no signs of return of spontaneous circulation (ROSC), go to **10** or **11**
- If ROSC, go to Post–Cardiac Arrest Care

© 2010 American Heart Association

CPR Quality ☐
- Push hard ($\geq$5 cm [2 inches]) and fast ($\geq$100/min) and allow complete chest recoil ☐
- Minimize interruptions in compressions ☐
- Avoid excessive ventilation
- Rotate compressor every 2 minutes
- If no advanced airway, 30:2 compression-ventilation ratio
- Quantitative waveform capnography
  - If P_{ETCO_2} <10 mm Hg, attempt to improve CPR quality
- Intra-arterial pressure
  - If relaxation phase (diastolic) pressure <20 mm Hg, attempt to improve CPR quality

Return of Spontaneous Circulation (ROSC)
- Pulse and blood pressure
- Abrupt sustained increase in P_{ETCO_2} (typically $\geq$40 mm Hg)
- Spontaneous arterial pressure waves with intra-arterial monitoring

Shock Energy
- **Biphasic:** Manufacturer recommendation (e.g., initial dose of 120-200 J); if unknown, use maximum available. Second and subsequent doses should be equivalent, and higher doses may be considered.
- **Monophasic:** 360 J

Drug Therapy
- **Epinephrine IV/IO Dose:** 1 mg every 3-5 minutes
- **Vasopressin IV/IO Dose:** 40 units can replace first or second dose of epinephrine
- **Amiodarone IV/IO Dose:** First dose: 300 mg bolus. Second dose: 150 mg.

Advanced Airway
- Supraglottic advanced airway or endotracheal intubation
- Waveform capnography to confirm and monitor ET tube placement
- 8-10 breaths per minute with continuous chest compressions

Reversible Causes ☐
- **H**ypovolemia
- **H**ypoxia
- **H**ydrogen ion (acidosis)
- **H**ypo-/hyperkalemia
- **H**ypothermia
- **T**ension pneumothorax
- **T**amponade, cardiac
- **T**oxins
- **T**hrombosis, pulmonary
- **T**hrombosis, coronary

159

Immediate Post–Cardiac Arrest Care Learning Station Checklist

Adult Immediate Post–Cardiac Arrest Care

1 Return of Spontaneous Circulation (ROSC)

2 ☐ Optimize ventilation and oxygenation
- Maintain oxygen saturation ≥94%
- Consider advanced airway and waveform capnography
- Do not hyperventilate

3 ☐ Treat hypotension (SBP <90 mm Hg)
- IV/IO bolus
- Vasopressor infusion
- Consider treatable causes
- 12-Lead ECG

4 Follow commands?

5 ☐ Consider induced hypothermia — No

6 ☐ STEMI OR high suspicion of **AMI** — Yes

7 ☐ Coronary reperfusion — Yes

8 ☐ Advanced critical care — No

Doses/Details

Ventilation/Oxygenation
Avoid excessive ventilation. Start at 10-12 breaths/min and titrate to target P_{ETCO_2} of 35-40 mm Hg. When feasible, titrate F_{IO_2} to minimum necessary to achieve SpO_2 ≥94%.

IV Bolus
1-2 L normal saline or lactated Ringer's. If inducing hypothermia, may use 4°C fluid.

Epinephrine IV Infusion:
0.1-0.5 mcg/kg per minute (in 70-kg adult: 7-35 mcg per minute)

Dopamine IV Infusion:
5-10 mcg/kg per minute

Norepinephrine IV Infusion:
0.1-0.5 mcg/kg per minute (in 70-kg adult: 7-35 mcg per minute)

☐ **Reversible Causes**
- **H**ypovolemia
- **H**ypoxia
- **H**ydrogen ion (acidosis)
- **H**ypo-/hyperkalemia
- **H**ypothermia
- **T**ension pneumothorax
- **T**amponade, cardiac
- **T**oxins
- **T**hrombosis, pulmonary
- **T**hrombosis, coronary

© 2010 American Heart Association

Bradycardia Learning Station Checklist

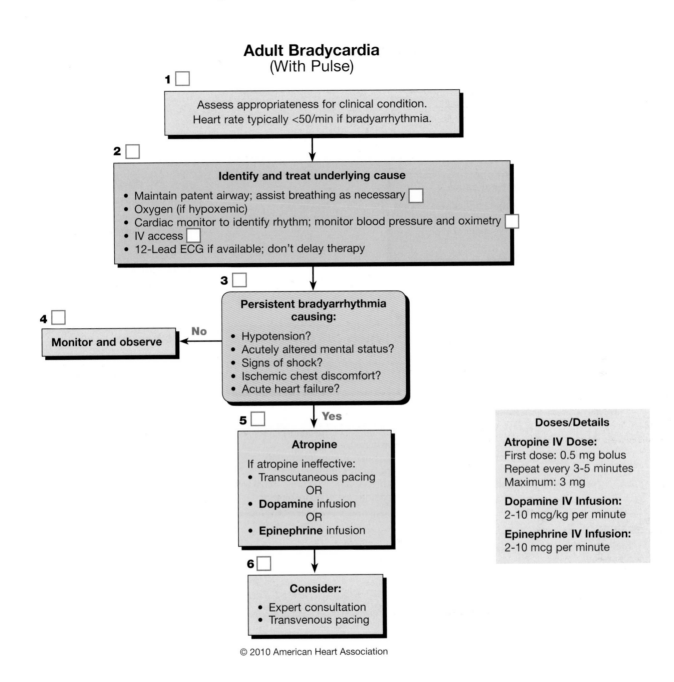

Adult Bradycardia
(With Pulse)

1 ☐

Assess appropriateness for clinical condition.
Heart rate typically <50/min if bradyarrhythmia.

2 ☐

Identify and treat underlying cause

- Maintain patent airway; assist breathing as necessary ☐
- Oxygen (if hypoxemic)
- Cardiac monitor to identify rhythm; monitor blood pressure and oximetry ☐
- IV access ☐
- 12-Lead ECG if available; don't delay therapy

3 ☐

Persistent bradyarrhythmia causing:

- Hypotension?
- Acutely altered mental status?
- Signs of shock?
- Ischemic chest discomfort?
- Acute heart failure?

No →

4 ☐

Monitor and observe

Yes

5 ☐

Atropine

If atropine ineffective:
- **Transcutaneous pacing**
  OR
- **Dopamine** infusion
  OR
- **Epinephrine** infusion

6 ☐

Consider:

- Expert consultation
- Transvenous pacing

Doses/Details

Atropine IV Dose:
First dose: 0.5 mg bolus
Repeat every 3-5 minutes
Maximum: 3 mg

Dopamine IV Infusion:
2-10 mcg/kg per minute

Epinephrine IV Infusion:
2-10 mcg per minute

© 2010 American Heart Association

Tachycardia Learning Station Checklist

Adult Tachycardia
(With Pulse)

1 ☐

Assess appropriateness for clinical condition.
Heart rate typically ≥150/min if tachyarrhythmia.

2 ☐

Identify and treat underlying cause

- Maintain patent airway; assist breathing as necessary ☐
- Oxygen (if hypoxemic)
- Cardiac monitor to identify rhythm; monitor blood pressure and oximetry ☐

3 ☐

Persistent tachyarrhythmia causing:

- Hypotension?
- Acutely altered mental status?
- Signs of shock?
- Ischemic chest discomfort?
- Acute heart failure?

Yes →

4 ☐

Synchronized cardioversion

- Consider sedation
- If regular narrow complex, consider adenosine

5 ☐   **No**

Wide QRS?
≥0.12 second

Yes →

6 ☐

- IV access and 12-lead ECG if available
- Consider adenosine only if regular and monomorphic
- Consider antiarrhythmic infusion
- Consider expert consultation

No

7 ☐

- IV access and 12-lead ECG if available
- Vagal maneuvers
- Adenosine (if regular)
- β-Blocker or calcium channel blocker
- Consider expert consultation

© 2010 American Heart Association

Doses/Details

Synchronized Cardioversion
Initial recommended doses:
- Narrow regular: 50-100 J
- Narrow irregular: 120-200 J biphasic or 200 J monophasic
- Wide regular: 100 J
- Wide irregular: defibrillation dose (NOT synchronized)

Adenosine IV Dose:
First dose: 6 mg rapid IV push; follow with NS flush.
Second dose: 12 mg if required.

Antiarrhythmic Infusions for Stable Wide-QRS Tachycardia

Procainamide IV Dose:
20-50 mg/min until arrhythmia suppressed, hypotension ensues, QRS duration increases >50%, or maximum dose 17 mg/kg given. Maintenance infusion: 1-4 mg/min. Avoid if prolonged QT or CHF.

Amiodarone IV Dose:
First dose: 150 mg over 10 minutes. Repeat as needed if VT recurs. Follow by maintenance infusion of 1 mg/min for first 6 hours.

Sotalol (not available in Canada) IV Dose:
100 mg (1.5 mg/kg) over 5 minutes. Avoid if prolonged QT.

2010 Guidelines for CPR and ECC Summary Table

Topic	2005 Guidelines	2010 Guidelines
Systematic Approach: BLS Survey	• A-B-C-D: Airway, Breathing, Circulation, Defibrillation • "Look, listen, and feel" for breathing and give 2 rescue breaths	• 1-2-3-4 **1. Check responsiveness.** **2. Activate the emergency response system and get an AED.** **3. Circulation:** Check the carotid pulse. If you cannot detect a pulse within 10 seconds, start CPR, beginning with chest compressions, immediately. **4. Defibrillation:** If indicated, deliver a shock with an AED or defibrillator.

Topic	2010 Guidelines	
BLS: High-Quality CPR	• A rate of **at least 100** chest compressions per minute • A compression depth of **at least 5 cm (2 inches)** in adults • Allowing complete chest recoil after each compression • Minimizing interruptions in compressions (10 seconds or less) • Switching providers about every 2 minutes to avoid fatigue • Avoiding excessive ventilation	
ACLS: Cardiac Arrest and Bradycardia Algorithms	• The *2010 Guidelines for CPR and ECC* simplifies the Cardiac Arrest Alogorithm and includes a circular algorithm. • The priority is the 2-minute continuous period of high-quality CPR and defibrillation. • All advanced interventions—including IV access, drug delivery, and advanced airways—should not interrupt chest compressions and shocks. Rather, they should be performed or administered strategically **after** the brief pause for defibrillation. • These actions continue until ROSC, when healthcare providers initiate post–cardiac arrest care protocols. • During cardiac arrest, providers should administer a vasopressor every 3 to 5 minutes. Epinephrine is commonly used, although vasopressin can replace the first or second dose of epinephrine. Regardless of the vasopressor given, one should be administered every 3 to 5 minutes. ACLS providers should administer amiodarone for refractory VF and VT. • The American Heart Association no longer recommends atropine for routine use in managing PEA or asystole. • For treatment of undifferentiated wide-complex tachycardia with regular rhythm, ACLS providers can consider adenosine in the initial treatment. • Atropine remains the first-line treatment for all symptomatic bradycardias, regardless of type. • For symptomatic bradycardia, the American Heart Association now recommends IV infusion of chronotropic agents as an equally effective alternative to external transcutaneous pacing when atropine is ineffective.	

(continued)

(continued)

Topic	2010 Guidelines
ACLS: Tachycardia– Synchronized Cardioversion	• The *2010 Guidelines for CPR and ECC* simplifies the Tachycardia Algorithm. • For cardioversion of unstable atrial fibrillation, the *2010 Guidelines for CPR and ECC* recommends that the initial biphasic energy dose be between 120 and 200 J. • For cardioversion of unstable SVT or unstable atrial flutter, the *2010 Guidelines for CPR and ECC* recommends that the initial biphasic energy dose be between 50 to 100 J. • Cardioversion with monophasic waveforms should begin at 200 J and increase in a stepwise fashion if not successful. • The *2010 Guidelines for CPR and ECC* also recommends cardioversion for unstable monomorphic VT, with an initial energy dose of 100 J. • If the initial shock fails, providers should increase the dose in a stepwise fashion.
ACLS: Post–Cardiac Arrest Care	A new section focusing on post–cardiac arrest care was introduced in the *2010 Guidelines for CPR and ECC*. Recommendations aimed at improving survival after ROSC include • Optimizing cardiopulmonary function and vital organ perfusion, especially to the brain and heart • Transporting out-of-hospital cardiac arrest patients to an appropriate facility with post–cardiac arrest care that includes acute coronary interventions, neurologic care, goal-directed critical care, and hypothermia • Transporting in-hospital cardiac arrest patients to a critical care unit capable of providing comprehensive post–cardiac arrest care • Identifying and treating the causes of the arrest and preventing recurrence • Considering therapeutic hypothermia to optimize survival and neurologic recovery in comatose patients • Identifying and treating acute coronary syndromes • Optimizing mechanical ventilation to minimize lung injury • Gathering data for prognosis • Assisting patients and families with rehabilitation services if needed **Critical actions for post–cardiac arrest care:** • Hemodynamic optimization, including a focus on treating hypotension • Acquisition of a 12-lead ECG • Induction of therapeutic hypothermia • Monitoring advanced airway placement and ventilation status with quantitative waveform capnography in intubated patients • Optimizing arterial oxygen saturation
ACLS: Managing the Airway	• The *2010 Guidelines for CPR and ECC* recommends using waveform capnography to monitor the amount of carbon dioxide exhaled by the patient and to verify placement of an endotracheal tube. • Cricoid pressure should not be used routinely during cardiac arrest. This technique is difficult to master and may not be effective for preventing aspiration. It may also delay or prevent placement of an advanced airway. • Agonal gasps are not effective breaths and should not be confused with normal breathing.
High-Quality Patient Care: Systems of Care	• Integrated systems of care should include community members, EMS, physicians, and hospitals.

ACLS Pharmacology Summary Table

Drug	Indications	Precautions/ Contraindications	Adult Dosage
Adenosine	• First drug for most forms of stable narrow-complex SVT. Effective in terminating those due to reentry involving AV node or sinus node • May consider for unstable narrow-complex reentry tachycardia while preparations are made for cardioversion • Regular and monomorphic wide-complex tachycardia, thought to be or previously defined to be reentry SVT • Does *not* convert atrial fibrillation, atrial flutter, or VT • Diagnostic maneuver: stable narrow-complex SVT	• Contraindicated in poison/drug-induced tachycardia or second- or third-degree heart block • Transient side effects include flushing, chest pain or tightness, brief periods of asystole or bradycardia, ventricular ectopy • Less effective (larger doses may be required) in patients taking theophylline or caffeine • Reduce initial dose to 3 mg in patients receiving dipyridamole or carbamazepine, in heart transplant patients, or if given by central venous access • If administered for irregular, polymorphic wide-complex tachycardia/VT, may cause deterioration (including hypotension) • Transient periods of sinus bradycardia and ventricular ectopy are common after termination of SVT • Safe and effective in pregnancy	**IV Rapid Push** • Place patient in mild reverse Trendelenburg position before administration of drug • Initial bolus of 6 mg given *rapidly* over 1 to 3 seconds followed by NS bolus of 20 mL; then elevate the extremity • A second dose (12 mg) can be given in 1 to 2 minutes if needed **Injection Technique** • Record rhythm strip during administration • Draw up adenosine dose and flush in 2 separate syringes • Attach both syringes to the IV injection port closest to patient • Clamp IV tubing above injection port • Push IV adenosine *as quickly as possible* (1 to 3 seconds) • While maintaining pressure on adenosine plunger, push NS flush *as rapidly as possible* after adenosine • Unclamp IV tubing
Amiodarone	Because its use is associated with toxicity, amiodarone is indicated for use in patients with life-threatening arrhythmias when administered with appropriate monitoring: • VF/pulseless VT unresponsive to shock delivery, CPR, and a vasopressor • Recurrent, hemodynamically unstable VT *With expert consultation* amiodarone may be used for treatment of some atrial and ventricular arrhythmias	***Caution:* Multiple complex drug interactions** • Rapid infusion may lead to hypotension • With multiple dosing, cumulative doses >2.2 g over 24 hours are associated with significant hypotension in clinical trials • Do not administer with other drugs that prolong QT interval (e.g., procainamide) • Terminal elimination is extremely long (half-life lasts up to 40 days)	**VF/VT Cardiac Arrest Unresponsive to CPR, Shock, and Vasopressor** • **First dose:** 300 mg IV/IO push • **Second dose (if needed):** 150 mg IV/IO push **Life-Threatening Arrhythmias** **Maximum cumulative dose:** 2.2 g IV over 24 hours. May be administered as follows: • **Rapid infusion:** 150 mg IV over first 10 minutes (15 mg per minute). May repeat rapid infusion (150 mg IV) every 10 minutes as needed • **Slow infusion:** 360 mg IV over 6 hours (1 mg per minute) • **Maintenance infusion:** 540 mg IV over 18 hours (0.5 mg per minute)

(continued)

Drug	Indications	Precautions/ Contraindications	Adult Dosage
Atropine Sulfate *Can be given via endotracheal tube*	• First drug for symptomatic sinus bradycardia • May be beneficial in presence of AV nodal block . Not likely to be effective for type II second-degree or third-degree AV block or a block in non-nodal tissue • Routine use during PEA or asystole is unlikely to have a therapeutic benefit • Organophosphate (e.g., nerve agent) poisoning: extremely large doses may be needed	• Use with caution in presence of myocardial ischemia and hypoxia. Increases myocardial oxygen demand • Avoid in hypothermic bradycardia • Will not be effective for infranodal (type II) AV block and new third-degree block with wide QRS complexes. (In these patients may cause paradoxical slowing. Be prepared to pace or give catecholamines) • Doses of atropine <0.5 mg may result in paradoxical slowing of heart rate	**Bradycardia (With or Without ACS)** • 0.5 mg IV every 3 to 5 minutes as needed, not to exceed total dose of 0.04 mg/kg (total 3 mg) • Use shorter dosing interval (3 minutes) and higher doses in severe clinical conditions **Organophosphate Poisoning** Extremely large doses (2 to 4 mg or higher) may be needed
Dopamine *IV infusion*	• Second-line drug for symptomatic bradycardia (after atropine) • Use for hypotension (SBP ≤70 to 100 mm Hg) with signs and symptoms of shock	• Correct hypovolemia with volume replacement before initiating dopamine • Use with caution in cardiogenic shock with accompanying CHF • May cause tachyarrhythmias, excessive vasoconstriction • Do not mix with sodium bicarbonate	**IV Administration** • Usual infusion rate is 2 to 20 mcg/kg per minute • Titrate to patient response; taper slowly
Epinephrine *Can be given via endotracheal tube* *Available in 1:10 000 and 1:1000 concentrations*	• **Cardiac arrest:** VF, pulseless VT, asystole, PEA • **Symptomatic bradycardia:** Can be considered after atropine as an alternative infusion to dopamine • **Severe hypotension:** Can be used when pacing and atropine fail, when hypotension accompanies bradycardia, or with phosphodiesterase enzyme inhibitor • **Anaphylaxis, severe allergic reactions:** Combine with large fluid volume, corticosteroids, antihistamines	• Raising blood pressure and increasing heart rate may cause myocardial ischemia, angina, and increased myocardial oxygen demand • High doses do not improve survival or neurologic outcome and may contribute to postresuscitation myocardial dysfunction • Higher doses *may* be required to treat poison/drug-induced shock	**Cardiac Arrest** • **IV/IO dose:** 1 mg (10 mL of 1:10 000 solution) administered every 3 to 5 minutes during resuscitation. Follow each dose with 20 mL flush, elevate arm for 10 to 20 seconds after dose • **Higher dose:** Higher doses (up to 0.2 mg/kg) may be used for specific indications (β-blocker or calcium channel blocker overdose) • **Continuous infusion:** Initial rate: 0.1 to 0.5 mcg/kg per minute (for 70-kg patient: 7 to 35 mcg per minute); titrate to response • **Endotracheal route:** 2 to 2.5 mg diluted in 10 mL NS **Profound Bradycardia or Hypotension** 2 to 10 mcg per minute infusion; titrate to patient response

(continued)

(continued)

Drug	Indications	Precautions/ Contraindications	Adult Dosage
Lidocaine *Can be given via endotracheal tube*	• Alternative to amiodarone in cardiac arrest from VF/VT • Stable monomorphic VT with preserved ventricular function • Stable polymorphic VT with normal baseline QT interval and preserved LV function when ischemia is treated and electrolyte balance is corrected • Can be used for stable polymorphic VT with baseline QT-interval prolongation if torsades suspected	• **Contraindication:** *Prophylactic* use in AMI is contraindicated • Reduce maintenance dose (not loading dose) in presence of impaired liver function or LV dysfunction • Discontinue infusion immediately if signs of toxicity develop	**Cardiac Arrest From VF/VT** • Initial dose: 1 to 1.5 mg/kg IV/IO • For refractory VF may give additional 0.5 to 0.75 mg/kg IV push, repeat in 5 to 10 minutes; maximum 3 doses or total of 3 mg/kg **Perfusing Arrhythmia** For stable VT, wide-complex tachycardia of uncertain type, significant ectopy: • Doses ranging from 0.5 to 0.75 mg/kg and up to 1 to 1.5 mg/kg may be used • Repeat 0.5 to 0.75 mg/kg every 5 to 10 minutes; maximum total dose: 3 mg/kg **Maintenance Infusion** 1 to 4 mg per minute (30 to 50 mcg/kg per minute)
Magnesium Sulfate	• Recommended for use in cardiac arrest only if torsades de pointes or suspected hypomagnesemia is present • Life-threatening ventricular arrhythmias due to digitalis toxicity • Routine administration in hospitalized patients with AMI is **not** recommended	• Occasional fall in blood pressure with rapid administration • Use with caution if renal failure is present	**Cardiac Arrest (due to Hypomagnesemia or Torsades de Pointes)** 1 to 2 g (2 to 4 mL of a 50% solution) diluted in 10 mL of D_5W IV/IO **Torsades de Pointes With a Pulse or AMI With Hypomagnesemia** • Loading dose of 1 to 2 g mixed in 50 to 100 mL of D_5W, over 5 to 60 minutes IV • Follow with 0.5 to 1 g per hour IV (titrate to control torsades)
Vasopressin *Can be given via endotracheal tube*	• May be used as alternative pressor to epinephrine in treatment of adult shock-refractory VF • May be useful alternative to epinephrine in asystole, PEA • May be useful for hemodynamic support in vasodilatory shock (e.g., septic shock)	• Potent peripheral vasoconstrictor. Increased peripheral vascular resistance may provoke cardiac ischemia and angina • Not recommended for responsive patients with coronary artery disease	**IV Administration** **Cardiac arrest:** One dose of 40 units IV/IO push may replace either first or second dose of epinephrine. Epinephrine can be administered every 3 to 5 minutes during cardiac arrest **Vasodilatory shock:** Continuous infusion of 0.02 to 0.04 units per minute

Glossary

A	
Acute	Having a sudden onset and short course
Acute myocardial infarction (AMI)	The early critical stage of necrosis of heart muscle tissue caused by blockage of a coronary artery
Advanced cardiovascular life support (ACLS)	Emergency medical procedures in which basic life support efforts of CPR are supplemented with drug administration, IV fluids, etc
Asystole	Absence of electrical and mechanical activity in the heart
Atrial fibrillation	In atrial fibrillation the atria "quiver" chaotically and the ventricles beat irregularly
Atrial flutter	Rapid, irregular atrial contractions due to an abnormality of atrial excitation
Atrioventricular block	A delay in the normal flow of electrical impulses that cause the heart to beat
Automated external defibrillator (AED)	A portable device used to restart a heart that has stopped

B	
Basic life support (BLS)	Emergency treatment of a victim of cardiac or respiratory arrest through cardiopulmonary resuscitation and emergency cardiovascular care
Bradycardia	Slow heartbeat, whether physiologically or pathologically

C	
Capnography	The measurement and graphic display of CO_2 levels in the airways, which can be performed by infrared spectroscopy
Cardiac arrest	Temporary or permanent cessation of the heartbeat
Cardiopulmonary resuscitation (CPR)	A basic emergency procedure for life support, consisting of mainly manual external cardiac massage and some artificial respiration
Coronary syndrome	A group of clinical symptoms compatible with acute myocardial ischemia (also called *coronary heart disease*)
Coronary thrombosis	The blocking of the coronary artery of the heart by a thrombus

E	
Electrocardiogram (ECG)	A test that provides a typical record of normal heart action
Encephalopathy	Degeneration of brain function. Also called *cephalopathy*, *cerebropathy*.
Endotracheal intubation	The passage of a tube through the nose or mouth into the trachea for maintenance of the airway
Esophageal detector device	A disposable tool used to verify proper endotracheal tube placement by using the anatomical differences between the trachea and esophagus
Esophageal-tracheal tube	A double-lumen tube with inflatable balloon cuffs that seal off the hypopharynx from the oropharynx and esophagus; used for airway management

H	
Hydrogen ion (acidosis)	The accumulation of acid and hydrogen ions or depletion of the alkaline reserve (bicarbonate content) in the blood and body tissues, decreasing the pH
Hyperkalemia	An abnormally high concentration of potassium ions in the blood. Also called *hyperpotassemia*.
Hypoglycemia	An abnormally low concentration of glucose in the blood
Hypokalemia	An abnormally low concentration of potassium ions in the blood. Also called *hypopotassemia*.
Hypothermia	A potentially fatal condition that occurs when body temperature falls below 95°F (35°C)
Hypovolemia	A decrease in the volume of circulating blood
Hypoxia	A deficiency of oxygen reaching the tissues of the body
I	
Intraosseous (IO)	Within a bone
Intravenous (IV)	Within a vein
M	
Mild hypothermia	When the patient's body temperature is between 90 and 95°F (32°C - 35°C)
Moderate hypothermia	When the patient's body temperature is between 86 and 90°F (30°C - 32°C)
N	
Nasopharyngeal	Pertaining to the nose and pharynx
O	
Oropharyngeal airway	A tube used to provide free passage of air between the mouth and pharynx
P	
Perfusion	The passage of fluid (such as blood) through a specific organ or area of the body (such as the heart)
Prophylaxis	Prevention of or protection against disease
Pulmonary edema	A condition in which fluid accumulates in the lungs
Pulseless electrical activity (PEA)	Continued electrical rhythmicity of the heart in the absence of effective mechanical function
R	
Recombinant tissue plasminogen activator (rtPA)	A clot-dissolving substance produced naturally by cells in the walls of blood vessels
S	
Severe hypothermia	When the patient's body temperature is <86°F (30°C)
Sinus rhythm	The rhythm of the heart produced by impulses from the sinoatrial node
Supraglottic	Situated or occurring above the glottis
Synchronized cardioversion	Uses a sensor to deliver a shock that is synchronized with a peak in the QRS complex

Syncope	A loss of consciousness over a short period of time, caused by a temporary lack of oxygen in the brain
T	
Tachycardia	Increased heartbeat, usually ≥100/min
Tamponade (cardiac)	A condition caused by accumulation of fluid between the heart and the pericardium, resulting in excess pressure on the heart. This impairs the heart's ability to pump sufficient blood.
Tension pneumothorax	Pneumothorax resulting from a wound in the chest wall which acts as a valve that permits air to enter the pleural cavity but prevents its escape
Thrombus	A blood clot formed within a blood vessel
U	
Unsynchronized shock	An electrical shock that will be delivered as soon as the operator pushes the SHOCK button to discharge the defibrillator. Thus, the shock can fall anywhere within the cardiac cycle.
V	
Ventricular fibrillation (VF)	Very rapid uncoordinated fluttering contractions of the ventricles
Ventricular tachycardia (VT)	A rapid heartbeat that originates in one of the lower chambers (ventricles) of the heart

Foundation Index